Okinawa's Complete Karate System—Isshin-Ryu

Okinawa's
Complete Karate System

**I
S
S
H
I
N
•
R
Y
U**

Michael
Rosenbaum

YMAA Publication Center
Boston, Mass. USA

YMAA Publication Center
Main Office
    4354 Washington Street
    Boston, Massachusetts, 02131
    1-800-669-8892 • www.ymaa.com • ymaa@aol.com

20191228

ISBN-13: 978-1-886969-91-9
ISBN-10: 1-886969-91-4

Publisher's Cataloging in Publication
(Prepared by Quality Books Inc.)

Rosenbaum, Michael, 1961-
        Okinawa's complete karate system : Isshin-ryu /
    Michael Rosenbaum. —1st ed.
        p. cm.
        Includes bibliographical references and index.
        LCCN: 00-106677
        ISBN: 1-886969-91-4

        1. Karate—Japan—Okinawa Island.   I. Title.

    GV1114.3.R67 2001   796.815'3
                                 QBI01-200149

Cover design by Richard Rossiter
Cover map courtesy www.lib.utexas.edu/Libs/PCL/Map collection
Text illustrations by the author
Edited by David Ganulan

Printed in USA.

To my wife Jennifer who has brought so much happiness into my life, my mother, Billie, who brought me into this life, and my mother-in-law Katie who is an inspiration to so many.

Contents

Foreword

Roots. Like everything else in life, the martial arts have roots. Each art, system, or style has its own history, lineage, and founder. This book is primarily about one martial art—Isshin-ryu karate: its history, its founder, its current state, and its future.

Michael Rosenbaum's approach is remarkably well balanced, for he offers sufficient detail to be highly informative yet presents the material in a readable format that holds the reader's attention. This makes the book beneficial not only to practitioners of Okinawan arts but also to students of other arts who are interested in simply broadening their perspective and appreciation of other styles.

Ultimately, the book's underlying message raises issues that go beyond any one art because, throughout its pages, we are reminded of the first tenets of martial art study—tenets that are are fundamental to the growth and development of all "martial" artists. First, we are reminded that martial arts are exactly that: martial. They were developed first and foremost for self-defense; be it for the battlefield soldier or ordinary citizen. That purpose should be obvious, but in our "kinder, gentler" day, it is often supplanted by the quest for self-development, perfection of character, or sporting competition.

The second tenet we are reminded of is the fact that the strongest and most enduring tradition in the martial arts—at least among those arts still claiming self-defense effectiveness—is change. Rosenbaum points out that Okinawan martial arts have always been works in progress, never reaching their founder's idea of perfection. This too should be self-evident, but alas, it is not. Far too many practitioners believe that preserving an art exactly as the master taught it (or, more correctly, as they perceived the master to have taught it), maintaining all the cultural rituals and trappings, preserves the effectiveness of the art as well. As well-intentioned as such preservationists are, they miss one very important point: preservation only works on dead subjects. A martial art is as alive as a living, breathing tiger; it is not a museum piece.

For me, what was surprising about this book was not the author's message—I agree with it wholeheartedly. Rather, it is that it was delivered by a "traditional" martial artist. There are other books out there that will tell you about Isshin-ryu karate; however, you will be hard pressed to find one that offers these kinds of insights into the real nature of karate as its founding masters intended it.

Bob Orlando

Bob Orlando is a martial arts instructor and the author of *Indonesian Fighting Fundamentals: The Brutal Arts of the Archipelago* (Paladin Press) and *Martial Arts America: A Western Approach to Eastern Arts* (North Atlantic Books/Frog Ltd.).

Preface

I began writing this book in 1987 and completed it in 1990. After finishing this manuscript it sat in my bookcase for close to 9 years until one day my wife encouraged me to try having it published. To her, David Ganulin, and YMAA Publication Center I am very grateful.

I'm always amazed at how fast time goes by. When this book is placed on the bookstore shelves it will have been 25 years since I began the study of Isshin-ryu Karate-Do. I still think of myself as a beginner, that skinny kid in a sweaty gi. What I find the most interesting about the passage of time is how much attitudes change. For instance, let me give the reader an example. Many martial artists today talk about how intense the Ultimate fighting contests are. I agree they are very demanding and intense, but in the dojo where I first began taking Isshin-ryu such intensity was commonly found in our sparring sessions. More than one dojo member had to be taken to the hospital for injuries sustained during sparring encounters. For the Isshin-ryu practitioner back then groin kicks were a way of life. This doesn't mean that there were not other schools that practiced in such a manner. The Bando practitioners were also noted for their aggressiveness in training even more so on some occasions. Edward Francisco and Allan Thompson would prove this more than once to me.

My outlook on the martial arts was developed as a teenager. I was very fortunate to have met some of the pioneers I write about in this book. I also consider myself lucky to have been instructed by some spectacular martial artists. They never achieved the level of fame as some of today's superstars but they are excellent martial artists nonetheless. People like Glenn Webb. One of the few men I've ever known who would shake the dojo floor from the force of his punches. Steve Trotter a walking dictionary of martial arts knowledge. Al White a man with shoulders that looked as wide as a Sherman tank and a fighting prowess to match. Maurice Mscarsa a man that could have easily overpowered any opponent yet had the grace and agility of a cat. There are many more who I fondly remember but have not the space to mention. My goal in writing this book was not to express it from the mainstream viewpoint but from that of the martial artist like those I have just mentioned. People who go to the dojo and practice for the sake of practice. I have attempted to present to the reader a picture of just where Isshin-ryu Karate evolved from, how it got to the United States and address some of the issues of its growth in America. The free enterprise system is a part of our American life style. There is nothing wrong with being paid for teaching martial arts. The problem occurs though when our ethics and standards of quality are replaced by the dollar sign. It seems we always want more of it and in turn look upon the martial arts as a vocation or quick way to earn extra income. The path to success in the martial arts is not through business management schools. The path to success in the martial arts is through hard work, sweat, and many years of practice. Once you have endured this time-honored path and come face to face with yourself then you may think about other ventures. Impatience is always the keystone of failure.

Michael Rosenbaum

Acknowledgements

I would like to thank the following people for making this book possible:

First and foremost, my wife, Jen who listens to my constant rambling about martial arts, and never complains about my early morning workouts.

Steve Condry, a long time friend who's done much leg work for me including typing and providing very insightful advice.

Chris Brock, my other long time friend and sparring partner. Those dull thuds from his punches on various parts of my body always bring me back to reality.

Allan Thompson and Ed Francisco, great friends, and even greater fighters with whom I've shared many laughs over the past ten years.

YMAA Publication Center for accepting this manuscript and making a dream come true.

Last, but not least, David Ganulin, for his editing of this manuscript and his conversations on martial arts.

Author's Note

   This text is not intended to be, in any form or fashion, the final say or a complete summary on Isshin-ryu karate or the Okinawan fighting arts. This is merely one person's views and ideals brought forth during his own development as a martial artist. Many who read the book may disagree with some of the facts and ideas presented. Some may even point out there are martial artists far more qualified than I to write on this subject. I am not in disagreement with any of these viewpoints, nor do I claim to be the world's foremost authority on Okinawan combative arts. I only hope that in reading this manuscript, some of these more experienced individuals may decide to put their knowledge down on paper to share with all of us. Until that time comes though, I hope this text may help some of us attain a deeper understanding of not only Isshin-ryu karate, but the martial arts as a whole.

   In today's society, Isshin-ryu karate, like many martial arts, finds itself in a very unique position, and at some very difficult crossroads. Isshin-ryu is one of the largest and fastest growing martial arts in North America. There are more people in the United States practicing Isshin-ryu today than there are Okinawan karate-ka combined. However, with all its growth and popularity, Isshin-ryu has come upon these crossroads seemingly unprepared. As Isshin-ryu as an organization continues to expand, it also grows apart with internal strife. As of this moment, there are six to ten different factions within the Isshin-ryu system, each one proclaiming to be following the true way of Tatsuo Shimabuku's (the founder) teachings. Organizations are not bad, but instead of each one proclaiming its way of karate as the "right way," we should try to break down the barriers separating us, overcome our egos, and work together to combine our knowledge so that all martial artists may benefit.

   Differences within Isshin-ryu can be used in very positive and imaginative ways, such as giving the martial artist standards of comparison during his own development. Without standards

of comparison, the practitioner will never have the variety needed to effectively judge if he or she is evolving or stagnating. A
standard of regulation is needed to keep a system's identity
intact, but it need not be enforced to the point where all forms
of individual creativity are eliminated. If this happens, the
process of evolution stops, and the system as a whole either
stagnates, dies out, or breaks off into factions that may be at
odds with one another. Isshin-ryu today needs to balance uniformity with individual creativity. Should this not happen and
our differences remain unresolved, then Isshin-ryu will continue
to grow apart.

In the middle of all these political and organizational confines there are a handful of individuals who will not allow
political bickering to interfere with their progression. By progression I mean the expansion of their knowledge and skills,
not the acquisition of rank, as many of today's martial artists
have become so obsessed with. These types of people are a
somewhat special breed. In earlier times they may have been
referred to as *ronin*, a term to describe samurai warriors who
claimed no loyalty to any figurehead or one who lost his master. Many of these types of teachers hold no standing in any
organization and could care less for rank or fame. The only
loyalty they hold is to perfecting their own skills and to the
practice of the martial arts. Organizations do not hamper
these people in their quest for knowledge, nor do particular
systems or even styles. All knowledge is useful to these individuals who may train in the confines of their backyard teaching
for little or no profit to small groups of devoted students.
Sometimes these individuals are shunned or blacklisted due to
dojo politics. This does not phase them however, because their
only goal is to practice the martial arts, learn, teach, and enjoy
themselves while doing so.

In today's title conscious society with progress commonly
being judged by trophies won and rank held, it is worth not-
ing these special individuals and their quest for martial perfection. They have become more important recently, especially
considering the quagmire that results when politics and ego
become motivating factors in studying a martial art. It is
sometimes hard to keep in mind that practicing a martial art is

an endless journey through a maze of constant change and evolution. Not only does this hold true for the individual, but also for the various systems and styles that help shape the state of martial arts in America. It will only benefit the arts as whole if, sometime during our own development, we stop and ask ourselves: Do we want to take shortcuts which will bestow short-lived moments of glory or should we continue on very rocky, well-worn path that will draw us closer to ourselves and mankind?

Postscript. The development of Okinawan martial arts was heavily influenced by both internal and external systems of Chinese fighting. An excellent source of research on this matter is Dr. Yang, Jwing-Ming's book *The Essence of Shaolin White Crane—Martial Power and Qigong.*

Dr Yang has over 40 years of experience in the martial arts and his book provides valuable insight into the origins of the Okinawan systems. As an Isshin-ryu Karate-Do practitioner with 25 years of experience I highly recommend *The Essence of Shaolin White Crane—Martial Power and Qigong* or any of the other quality books by YMAA Publication Center.

Michael Rosenbaum
February 8, 2001

Introduction

The subject matter of this text is focused upon Tatsuo Shimabuku's system of Isshin-ryu karate, the 'one heart-one mind' way. To completely understand Isshin-ryu, or any form of Okinawan fighting art, it helps to examine the history from which it came, the strong relationships between Okinawan fighting styles (*ryu*), and the early cultural and political relationships between China and Okinawa.

When examining a system, it is sometimes helpful to look at what was occurring historically when the system was conceived. For instance, the Ryukyuan fighting arts had been evolving since the ninth century, but there were perhaps two key events that helped spur their expansion. One was the Okinawan government's fifteenth-century ban on private ownership of weapons. The second was the conquest of Okinawa by Japan in the seventeenth century during which time Japanese forces forbade ownership of any weapons or practice of any martial art.

These two milestones helped spur the development of Te as an effective means of self-defense and a tool to use in insurgent activities against the Japanese. From that conflict eventually came what is now known as Okinawan karate and Kobudo. Whether it be Shuri-te, Naha-te, Goju-ryu, or Shorin-ryu their immediate roots and spark of conception can be traced back to that one period in Okinawan history, with many of their paths crossing frequently along the way.

In analyzing Okinawan systems, it is very hard to find a completely pure system of Okinawan karate. In using the term "pure," I refer to a style that has only come under influence from Shuri-te, Naha-te, or Tomari-te. (*Te* means "hand" and was used in conjunction with geographical locations. It was also used with a person's name to describe systems of the day. For instance Shuri-te denoted fighting systems developed around the city of Shuri. Shimabuku-te meant Shimabuku's system.) One reason for the influences one system had on another is Okinawa's small size. The three regions from which many of the fighting arts evolved were within walking distance of one another. It is not uncommon to find influence from all three systems upon any given style of Okinawan karate. For instance, the Shobayashi-ryu branch of Shorin-ryu karate is linked directly to early Shuri-te fighting methods. However, Chotoku Kyan, Shobayashi-ryu's founder, also studied with Matsumora Kosaku. Kosaku was a leading Tomari-te practitioner and from him, Kyan brought some Tomari-te technique into his Shorin-ryu. This also proves true for Isshin-ryu, which has a collection of both Shuri-te and Naha-te kata.

All Okinawan fighting systems have what are considered to be core techniques and principles, but many of these may also be found in other forms of Ryukyu fighting systems. What usually distinguishes one system from another, in many cases, is the significance placed upon a certain number of these central techniques and principles.

It is very hard when you start analyzing a style's lineage against the background of the Okinawan fighting arts. It is important to keep in mind that each style began as one person's teachings and interpretations organized into a system that they felt was efficient and worthy of use in combat. The founders were a fascinating group of men and this only helped contribute to the rich amalgam of Okinawan arts we have today.

CHAPTER 1

The Evolution of Okinawan Te and Karate-Jutsu

The Ryukyu Islands stretch from the southern tip of Kyushu, Japan, 735 miles southeast to Taiwan. Considering their location, it is easy to see how these islands have been a port of call for sailing vessels through the centuries. Okinawa is the largest of all the Ryukyuan islands and its name literally means 'a rope in the offing.' It has commonly been described as the melting pot of the orient. Ryukyuan culture holds traces of many other Asian societies including Chinese, Japanese, Malaysian, and Thai.

There is a long history of warfare in Ryukyuan culture, from the second century up to the present day. Prior to the second century, Ryukyuan culture was primarily Neolithic. The means by which the Okinawans produced and utilized weapons were very crude and any advances made by the Okinawans at this point would have been from Chinese influences. By the ninth and tenth centuries, Okinawa had become an island divided into three kingdoms, each swarming with marauding bands of thugs and people who would commit any atrocity to achieve power. It was during this turbulent time in Ryukyuan history that survivors of the great Taira-Minamoto wars began making their way to Okinawa. These people sought refuge from a horrible conflict that had encompassed the entire Japanese mainland. They also brought to Okinawa many of the weapons and martial skills used during those wars.

Around the beginning of the eleventh century, Zen Buddhism was introduced to Okinawan society by Buddhist monks. Some of these monks had been exposed to Shaolin systems of fighting. Even though Buddhism would not play a

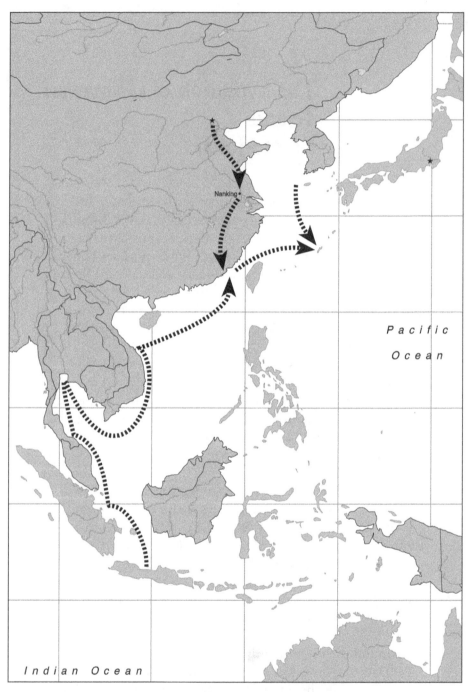

Nanking

Pacific

Ocean

Indian Ocean

East Asian trade routes. These are possible routes that
fighting techniques could have traveled to Okinawa.

major role in the development of Okinawan fighting arts, the monks' knowledge of Shaolin boxing systems would. At a later period in Ryukyuan history when relations with China became even stronger, a much larger variety of Chinese systems and techniques would make their way to Okinawa.

By 1352, the three kingdoms of Okinawa had been united under one ruling government and trade with other Asian countries began. Official Chinese-Okinawan relations were established in 1372. Soon after, Chinese priests, doctors, teachers, and military began arriving in Okinawa. It was during this time that fighting arts from other countries such as Thailand, Java, and Indonesia began making their way to the Ryukyu Islands. Chinese communities were also established in the towns of Shuri and Naha. In return, Okinawans were allowed to establish a community in what was then the Chinese capital city of Chuan Chou. In spite of the Chinese fighting systems already present, the Okinawans were busy developing fighting arts based upon their own findings. Not only did they include Chinese methods of combat, but also other Asian systems which already made their way to the island kingdom. The Okinawans referred to their methods of fighting as Tode, and the systems were noted for having hard, closed-handed, thrusting-type techniques. Many of these characteristics can still be seen in Okinawan karate today. The Isshin-ryu straight punch is considered by some as an offshoot of these techniques. The Tode systems relied heavily on physical dexterity and very aggressive offensive strategies to defeat an opponent.

The vast majority of Okinawan fighting methods at this time lacked the finesse and sophistication of their contemporary Chinese systems. Tode movements were noted for being bold and aggressive. This was very much in contrast to many Chinese systems of fighting, which were of a softer nature. The Chinese relied more upon open-handed blocking techniques with very subtle shifting movements. Their systems placed great emphasis upon body positioning, footwork, and angular and circular methods of movement. In later years, when Chinese influences became stronger and more apparent in Okinawan fighting arts, the Tode methods would still remain. It would be some time before circular stepping patterns, open-handed techniques, and other softer methods became integrated into the Okinawan fighting arts.

In 1479 the Okinawan government forbade private ownership of all weapons. This had the natural effect of creating an even greater interest in the development of empty-handed methods of combat by the Okinawans. It was not long after that the principle of *Temeshi-wari* was developed and practiced by Okinawan martial artists. Temeshi-wari refers to hardening the body, and involves developing calluses on certain areas that are used for striking and blocking. Some of these areas include the practitioner's knuckles, edge of the hand, shins, forearms, and toes. Some Okinawans developed this principle to such a degree that they were capable of punching through lacquered bamboo armor.

By 1600 relations between Okinawa and China had solidified. The Chinese communities on Okinawa were thriving, yet the Chinese and Okinawan fighting systems still remained fairly distinct. In 1609 Japanese forces invaded and eventually conquered Okinawa. Although an occupied land, the people of Okinawa remained very self-reliant and proud. Almost immediately they launched a campaign of guerrilla warfare against the Japanese. Strange as it may seem, the occupying Japanese still allowed the Okinawans to conduct trade with China, and travel between the two countries was unrestricted. Free travel and trade allowed many notable Chinese martial artists to journey to Okinawa. A number of these martial practitioners would later prove to play a major role in the development of Okinawan fighting arts.

There were many notable Okinawans who traveled to China as well. While abroad, they studied the various systems of Chinese boxing that included both the internal and external forms of the northern and southern systems. Although some of the Okinawans who journeyed to China stayed only months, others spent years there studying Chinese fighting methods before returning to Okinawa. Some of the more notable Okinawans to train in China were Chatan Yara, Sakugawa, and Kanryo Higashionna (sometimes written 'Higaonna.') Yara studied the staff and twin sword forms of fighting extensively. Sakugawa was Bushi Matsumora's sensei, and Higashionna was Miyagi Chojun's sensei. It was Miyagi who later founded another popular style of Okinawan karate called Goju-ryu. Some people believe that, at one point in time, Tatsuo Shimabuku, Isshin-ryu's founder, also journeyed to China to further his knowledge of the martial arts.

From 1611 to 1810, there were few written records of Okinawan fighting. This was due to the band of secrecy placed around the art by its practitioners. One of the most amazing things about the Okinawan martial arts during this period is that the Japanese never found out who the Tode instructors were, or where the training was being conducted. What is known about the early development of Tode is that the sole objective and focus of this martial art was to kill. It was not uncommon to hear of unarmed practitioners facing off against armed samurai in combat. The Okinawan's martial arts could be considered their major weapon in waging their guerrilla campaign against the occupying Japanese forces. By 1629 the Okinawan Tode and Chinese systems of boxing present on the island had combined. The resulting system from this combination was to be known as Te which translates as "hand," and is widely regarded as modern karate's forefather.

One should keep in mind that although quite a number of Okinawans went to China where they studied Chinese fighting arts extensively, there were also many others who were, first and foremost, guerrilla fighters. These were warriors looking for techniques that were effective, easy to learn, and could be applied to combat almost immediately. In their search for these types of techniques, the Okinawans omitted from their Chinese studies aesthetic qualities and advanced principles which were believed not to be practical, or else would take too long to perfect. (This process was to be repeated and taken one step further by Shimabuku in his founding of Isshin-ryu years later.) Due to the Okinawans reluctance to utilize animal forms, and earlier Tode influences upon Okinawan fighting arts, it is easy to see why many Okinawan systems of karate appear to be rigid and linear in nature when compared to Chinese methods of boxing.

Early in the seventeenth century the Japanese imposed a

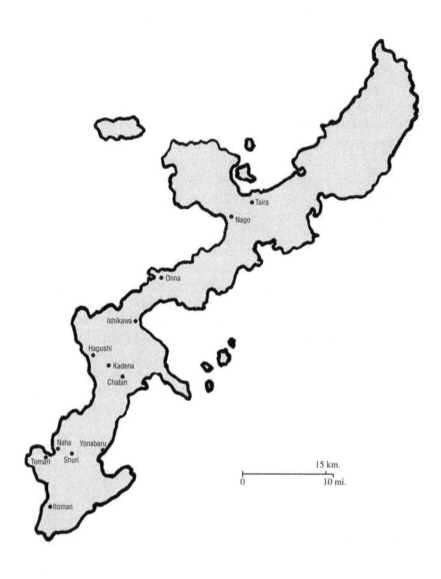

Map of Okinawa.

ban on the ownership of weapons. Te practitioners began developing their own, armed forms of fighting in conjunction with the development of unarmed methods. The Okinawans applied principles and techniques learned from other armed systems of combat to simple farming implements indigenous to their society. This system of armed combat that resulted came to be known as *Kobudo*. Along with Kobudo came the development of three distinct fighting arts from the original Te system. Each was named after the region or town in which its development took place. These systems were known as Shuri-te, which evolved around Shuri, Naha-te from Naha, and Tomari-te from Tomari.

Shuri-te systems emphasized the external, harder aspects of combat. It is said to have been primarily offensive in nature and stressed agility and quickness in movement. Shuri-te was heavily influenced by Shaolin methods of boxing and would later on come to be known as Shorin-ryu. This name refers to a small pine forest in Fukien province where one of the Shaolin systems of fighting originated. Since this name change, five forms of Shorin-ryu have come into being. They are the Matsumura-seito, founded by Hohan Soken; the Kobayashi-ryu or 'young forest style;' the Shobayashi-ryu or 'small forest style' developed by Chotoku Kyan; the Matsubayashi-ryu or 'pine forest style;' and the Shorinji-ryu. Traditionally Shuri-te utilized 14 empty-handed kata. They are Ananko, Chinte, Chinto, Seisan, Jion, Kusanku, Naihanchi, Neiseishi, Patsai, Pinan, Sochin, Ueshishi, and Unsu.

The methods of Te developed in Naha were sometimes referred to as Shorei-ryu. Naha-te was influenced more by internal methods of boxing such as Pa Kua and Hsing-I. Naha-te techniques tended to more defensive in nature, incorporating grappling and throwing techniques that had not been widely used in other systems of Okinawan Te. Naha-te movements are characterized by firm, forceful motions, but the system is noted for its practice of Sanchin—a controlled breathing exercise that incorporates dynamic tension. Sanchin is also known as 'The Three Conflicts' or 'Three Levels Breathing' kata. The three levels refer to the upper, middle, and lower areas of the body where dynamic tension and deep breathing are concentrated

From Naha-te evolved Goju-ryu. Goju-ryu, meaning 'hard-soft way' was founded by Chojun Miyagi who was also one of Shimabuku's instructors. Miyagi formalized the principles and techniques of Naha-te into modern day Goju. The style utilizes Kururumfa, Pechurin, Saifa, Sanchin, Sanseiryu, Seipai, Seisan, Seiuchin, Shisoochin, and Tensho katas.

Another system of karate strongly associated with Naha-te is Uechi-ryu. Uechi-ryu's lineage is probably more directly related to Chinese boxing methods than other Okinawan forms of Te. Its founder, Kanbun Uechi, who traveled to China in 1897, did much of Uechi-ryu's development outside of Okinawa. While in China, he studied a system called Pangai-noon and it was from this system that Uechi-ryu eventually evolved. Uechi's son, Kanyei, took over as head of the system when his father died in 1947. Uechi-ryu's kata are Kanchin, Kanshiwa, Kanshu, Sanchin, Sanseryu, Sechin, and Seiryu.

The Te developed in the Tomari area tended to be somewhat a mixture of both Naha and Shuri methods. Tomari-te stressed both internal and external aspects of Chinese methods. Tomari-te's ranks have held such notables as Matsumora Kosaku, Kuba Koho, Yamazota Kiki, Chotoku Kyan, and Motobu Choki, another of Tatsuo Shimabuku's instructors. One of the most recognized systems to come out of Tomari-te is Okinawan Kempo, founded by Shigeru Nakamura. Nakamura's system is a mixture of all three forms of Te. The kata within Okinawan Kempo are Ananko, Chinto, Kusanku, Naihanchi, Neiseichi, Patsai, Sanchin, Seisan and Wansu. (Isshin-ryu utilizes Seisan, Seiuchin, Naihanchi, Wansu, Chinto, Kusanku, Sanchin, and Sunsu, a kata developed by Tatsuo Shimabuku. Traditionally Isshin-ryu doesn't utilize Pinan kata.)

Although all three forms of Te differed in their approach to combat, they had one thing in common. All advocated the concept of movement from a natural body position. Te's combative sphere is not as extensive as that of the Bujutsu (Japanese arts of war) forms, nor is the mental discipline that is instilled in Bujutsu to be found in Okinawan Te.

The Bujutsu cover many areas and methods of armed and unarmed combat. These include *Ken-jutsu* or swordsmanship, *Kyu-jutsu,* bow and arrow methods, *Bo-jutsu* or staff techniques, and *Senjo-jutsu,* the art of tactics and strategy. In contrast, the Okinawan forms of combat were developed largely by civilians—not professional soldiers like the samurai. The scope of Okinawan methods concentrated more on empty handed techniques and utilizing the weapons available to them such as farming tools like the tonfa, kama, and sai. Traditionally, these implements are not included in the Japanese Bujutsu systems.

After the Meiji restoration in 1868, Japan forbade the practice of any martial art on Okinawa. From 1845 to 1941, Okinawa underwent Japanese assimilation and in 1875 Japanese occupation forces were removed from Okinawa. By this time the island kingdom was considered a sovereign state of Japan. The practice of Te was still conducted in secrecy, and it was during this era that Japanese systems 'martial ways' *(Budo)* were first introduced to Okinawa. Styles such as Kendo and Judo picked up a great many followers on the island. Later on the Okinawans would organize teams and compete against the Japanese. The impact Japanese Budo had on Okinawan Te systems however, was not very strong.

One of the most significant years in modern Okinawan history was 1903, when the first public demonstrations of Te were given. So impressed were governing officials that they allowed Te to be taught in public schools as a form of physical education. However, what was taught would not be the deadly combative form of fighting used in years past against Japanese forces. Instead this form was modified and many of the com-bative aspects were removed and replaced with concepts of a more sporting nature. One of Okinawa's finest Te masters, Itosu Yasutsune, helped bring the art into the public school systems. Not long after its introduction into the public schools, another historic change came about in its evolution.

Prior to formalization of the three Te systems, Okinawan fighting arts were not organized into styles. Instead, each method was recognized by the master who taught his own form. It was during this time when the term *kara-te* meaning

'Tang Hand Fist' came to be. Kara-te was used in a generic fashion to describe the various methods, for instance Matsumura Kara-te Matsumura's method of Te.

In 1903 the term *kara* was used once again in describing Okinawan fighting systems. Instead of simply being called Te, the name was changed to Karate-jutsu. The old ideogram representing *kara* was chosen because it symbolized the Tang dynasty—an era in which much knowledge of Chinese fighting methods was brought to Okinawa. The original ideogram that represented Te, (hand) was used to recognize the earlier Okinawan methods of combat. Jutsu was taken from the Japanese because it meant 'art,' a term used when describing arts or methods of conducting warfare. The end result of this terminology was *karate-jutsu,* or 'China Hand Art.' As cleverly as they had concealed Te for so many years, the Okinawans also managed to pay respect to three different cultures yet at the same time establish their own martial arts identity. Today there are estimated to be over 200 karate dojos on Okinawa. The major systems of Okinawan karate recognized today are Kobayashi-ryu, (Shorin-ryu) Matsubashi-ryu, (Shorin-ryu) Shobayashi-ryu, (Shorin-ryu) Goju-ryu, Isshin-ryu, Uechi-ryu and Okinawan Kempo.

The concept of Do and Karate's Introduction to Japan. In 1922 the Japanese Ministry of Education asked Okinawan karate-jutsu leaders to send an expert to demonstrate the art on the Japanese mainland. The man picked by the Okinawans was Gichin Funakoshi, a Shuri-te stylist who had studied under both Itosu and Azato. Funakoshi, the founder of Shotokan, is considered by many to be the father of Japanese karate. He is also noted for popularizing the change of the *kara* ideogram from one representing 'China' to one implying 'emptiness.' Karate now went from meaning 'China Hand Art' to 'Empty Hand Art.'

Funakoshi's change brought great protest from Okinawan practitioners. Many interpreted this to mean there were no weapons in Okinawan karate, something far from true since Kobudo had always played a major role in the Okinawan fighting arts. This was not what Funakoshi referred to when he changed the ideogram's meaning. Instead he was making reference to the spiritual aspects of karate, the emptying of oneself of all egotistical tendencies. Later on in Funakoshi's career, his efforts would enable some of the emerging Japanese karate systems of the time to be officially recognized as part of the Japanese Budo.

It was just prior to this time that some of the harsher overtones in Okinawan karate were being replaced. Until this point in time, Te systems were basically combative and very physical in nature. In 1926 Higashonna and Itosu began stressing a form of spiritual discipline in the practice of Te. This discipline would be used as a means to resolve conflict within one's life. The karate practitioner would train to react calmly and rationally to any given situation—combative or non-combative, spiritual as well as physical. This philosophy placed emphasis more on spiritual development, much as a form of Budo would.

Japanese Budo forms had been in existence for quite some time, but for the Okinawans, this change of focus in their art caused quite a bit of controversy. A 'Do's' emphasis is on self-development first with combative means and measures considered secondary. In contrast, a Jutsu art like *Aiki-jutsu* or *Ken-jutsu* focuses primarily upon combat. Most forms of Japanese Bujutsu were practiced by military personnel for use in combat. Their primary method of training was kata and it was generally agreed that Bujutsu techniques were far too dangerous for use in free sparring. The Budo counterparts however, systems like Kendo and Aikido were practiced by commoners for self-development and self-discipline, placing emphasis upon contest where contestants did utilize free sparring methods. The Budo systems modified their techniques to allow for use in competition. Many Okinawans felt this new emphasis would turn their karate into a form of organized sport. Some practitioners continued to train as they always had. Others however, agreed with Higashionna and Itosu's beliefs. It was during this time that free sparring methods first began being used in Okinawan karate.

Although many systems began placing emphasis upon the philosophical aspects, early Te influences were still present. Unlike many forms of Japanese Budo, the Okinawan's technique stayed combative by nature with kata remaining the dominant method of practice. Even Funakoshi, who stressed that his form of karate was a "Do" form, strictly enforced the rule within his teachings that karate was not a sport. It was an art for self-development and self-defense and that the practice of kata was true karate. This philosophy can also be seen in some of Funakoshi's top students like Nakayama, Yoshida, and Otsuka—the founder of Wado-ryu karate.

Gichin Funakoshi is by far the most recognized Okinawan for his efforts of introducing karate-jutsu to Japan. He was not however the only Okinawan to instruct the Japanese in the ways of Okinawan karate-jutsu. There were others, like Kenwa Mabuni who studied both Shuri-te and Naha-te. Mabuni later founded the Shito-ryu system. Choki Motobu and Chojun Miyagi are two other Okinawans who also went to Japan where their exploits gained fame. These are just a few of many Okinawans who helped lay the foundation for numerous Japanese systems of karate.

There are at least 100 styles of Japanese karate today. Some are considered to be "quasi-martial" forms by various Okinawan practitioners. One reason is the emphasis placed upon physical education and sporting competition by some Japanese systems. Okinawan karate-ka feel that self-defense takes a secondary role in many systems of Japanese karate. Many of these outlooks have no sound basis and can be attributed to martial rivalry.

Unlike traditional Okinawan forms of karate-jutsu, where Kobudo and karate go hand-in-hand, this is not the case with many Japanese systems, who instead tend to stress more empty-handed techniques. Among Japanese karate systems that do incorporate weapon arts within their teachings, it is not uncommon to see Kendo or some other Japanese weapons system being practiced in place of Kobudo.

Japanese karate today has been strongly influenced by other Japanese Budo. It is very common to see mixtures of the two. For instance the unification of Jujitsu and Karate became Wado-ryu. The major systems of Japanese karate today are Shotokan, from Gichin Funakoshi, Shito-ryu from Kenwa Mabuni, Wado-ryu from Otsuka, Japanese Goju-ryu founded by "The Cat" Yamaguchi, and Kyokushin by Mas Oyama.

In today's society we often find that the traditional boundaries of geography, race, or religion which once kept systems apart are quickly being overcome. This is also true in Japan today. When one analyzes the Okinawan and Japanese forms of karate it is helpful to keep this fact in mind, especially when trying to define what was originally an integral part of the system in comparison to what has been added in recent years. Many ultra-traditional practitioners are now accepting that it is okay to borrow knowledge, especially if that knowledge is useful. This also holds true in Isshin-ryu where it is not uncommon for the teachings of one dojo to differ from another.

Like Kung Fu, the word 'karate' has become a generic term associated with any form of fighting that makes use of hand and foot techniques. Even American sport systems, which at best could only be considered quasi-martial arts, fall under the heading of karate. Today karate not only covers Okinawan and Japanese systems, but also Korean, Chinese, and even Burmese fighting arts. In terms of Japanese and Okinawan karate today, differences distinguishing the two are still present, but not quite so defined as they once were.

CHAPTER 2

The Evolution of Okinawan Kobudo

Although Te is generally used to describe all Okinawan forms of combat prior to 1900, the Okinawans did not restrict their development of fighting systems only to unarmed methods. In most instances Te practitioners were versed in both armed and unarmed methods of combat. The evolution and development of Okinawan Kobudo parallels that of Okinawan Karate-Do. Kobudo literally means 'ancient martial ways,' a term that could be used in describing all original forms of Okinawan fighting arts.

Kobudo, like Okinawan karate, was also heavily influenced by Chinese fighting arts. One of the earliest influences on Okinawan Kobudo can be traced back to A.D. 517, when a Zen priest named Daruma Daishi formalized both staff and short sword techniques. One of the biggest single influences on Okinawan Kobudo came during the Ming Dynasty when the existing Chinese staff forms (some of which were handed down from Daruma) underwent a series of refinements. Soon afterwards these same staff techniques were taught to the Okinawans. Their interests in armed forms of fighting had been spurred on by laws preventing them from owning any weapon. To compensate for this, the Okinawans began taking techniques and principles from Chinese weapons systems and applied them to implements indigenous to their own society. In most cases these implements were simply farming tools of the day. For instance nunchuakus were originally used as rice flails and the tonfa's original function was as a millstone handle.

To fully envision the Okinawan fighting arts, picture a circle. One half is comprised of empty handed methods or Te, and the other is made up of armed methods of fighting or Kobudo. Both are separate systems within their own right, but

the two are integral parts of a whole with interlocking principles. Like a bicycle's wheels, they are independent yet linked
together by the same frame that complements each other.
Many styles of Okinawan karate are organized in this fashion.
For instance, of the 14 original kata in Isshin-ryu, six are
Kobudo kata. Although considered separate fighting arts, on
some occasions the two systems techniques and principles will
overlap. This is illustrated by the fact that it was a fairly common practice for Okinawan Te practitioners to perform their
empty-handed kata with weapons such as the sai or tonfa. In
some instances, Kobudo weapons are considered merely extensions of the hands while on other occasions distinctions are
made between the two.

A prime example of this for the Isshin-ryu stylist would be
the Kusanku and Chatan Yara sai katas. The Kusanku sai techniques overlap its empty-handed version's techniques. On the
other hand, Chatan Yara sai kata is basically a weapons kata
native to Okinawa Kobudo and has no empty-handed coun-
terpart. The practice of utilizing Kobudo weapons while performing empty-handed kata was done primarily with the sai,
tonfa and kama— weapons that were not very hard to adapt
to the kata. Although it can be done, this practice is not very
common with Bo (staff) techniques. This is largely due to the
weapon's nature. It is not unheard of to perform Bo kata
empty-handed and some karate-ka refer to this practice as the
Okinawan's own brand of tai chi. Kobudo's influence, or half
of the sphere that makes up the Okinawan fighting arts, can
be divided into three categories.

The first is the practice of Kobudo as an art within itself.
Many people consider the weapons forms as part of the empty-
handed systems. This is not true. Kobudo is a martial art within
its own right and to make such an assertion is to lose sight of
Kobudo's true perspective. There is also an extremist view taken
towards maintaining Kobudo's identity by some practitioners.
Those who focus only on weapons may find themselves weak in
the empty-handed aspects of the arts. He may soon arrive at a
point where he cannot function as a combatant without the use
of a weapon. One goal of the Okinawan fighting systems is to
develop complete warriors—practitioners versed in both armed
and unarmed methods of combat.

The second category can be classified as Kobudo's influence upon the empty-handed methods of Okinawan fighting arts. Some of the more advanced theories found within empty-handed methods were either taken directly from Kobudo, or were heavily influenced by Kobudo technique. For instance, quite a few techniques in the Okinawan karate arsenal deal with attacking the opponent's limbs. Isshin-ryu karate utilizes the theory that every empty-handed block can also be used as a strike. Attacking an opponent's limbs is a theory common to Kobudo and is something that can be seen in the empty-handed methods.

The third category is the utilization of weapons. In this mode, weapons become simply an extension of one's hands. When utilized in this fashion the Kobudo and Te techniques overlap. This can become a very dangerous practice for unskilled practitioners. In empty-handed fighting, combatants have designated target areas and certain portions of their bodies where blows can be sustained. This is not true with armed methods of combat where any area of an opponent's body is considered a target and if struck the results can be devastating. One example of this for Isshin-ryu practitioners is the Kusanku sai kata. Depending on which version is practiced, there are very little if any kicking techniques utilized. The rationale being that to kick from a distance at an opponent who was armed with staff or sword would more than likely result with a broken or amputated leg.

The techniques and principles that make up Okinawan Kobudo made their way to Okinawa in very much the same manner as empty-handed techniques did. Kobudo, like Te, also had its share of famous practitioners. In many cases they were the same person.

Perhaps one of the more famous Okinawan Kobudo practitioners was 'Yara' or Chatan Yara as he is more commonly known. Yara spent twenty years in China studying the martial arts and mastered both staff and short sword methods of fighting. Not only was he proficient with the staff and short swords, but he was also an accomplished Hsing-I practitioner. Yara is said to be one of the first people to introduce the principles of chi (internal energy) to Okinawan fighting arts. From

Yara's teachings Okinawan Kobudo has the Chatan Yara bo and sai katas.

Sakugawa also taught both Te and Kobudo. He began his study of the martial arts under a monk named Takahara Pechin and went on to study with Kusanku, a Chinese envoy. Later in his career Sakugawa journeyed to China where he furthered his knowledge of the martial arts. Sakugawa's most notable contributions to Okinawan martial arts are the bo (staff) Sakugawa No Kon and Kusanku katas. One of Sakguwa's most notable students was Donchi Ginowan, a man noted for his expertise in the sai and bo. Ginowan's skill was supposedly flawless and he's legendary in Okinawan Kobudo. Still another influential teacher was Chinen of Yamane-ryu. Chinen was a bo specialist who developed the Shushi No Kun, Ogusuku No Kun, and Gyaku No Kun bo katas. Notice that on many occasions, the suffix 'No Kun' used in conjunction with a bo kata's name. This term was used by Chinese martial artists during the Ming dynasty when describing staff fighting techniques. In an effort to pay homage to the Chinese from whom the Okinawans gained much knowledge of staff techniques, they included the suffix in the kata's name.

One of the more notable bo masters of Okinawan Kobudo was Sueishi. Born to a prominent samurai family in Shuri, he also ventured to China to expand his knowledge of the martial arts. Sueishi was well versed in all of the Kobudo weapons systems, but he was especially noted for his bo skills. Sueishi developed the Sueishi No Kon and Shoun No Kon bo katas.

Shinken Taira is one of the more well known Kobudo practitioners in this century. Taira studied Kobudo under Mouden Yabiku and karate with Gichin Funakoshi. Taira opened his first dojo in Ikaho City, where he taught both Karate and Kobudo. Later he would move to Naha, Okinawa and establish a Kobudo dojo there. Taira founded the Society for Promotion and Preservation of the Ryukyuan Martial Arts, and instructed such notables as Fumio Demura, Tatsuo Shimabuku and Motokatsu Inoue.

Kobudo was developed around several weapons, all of which were originally farming implements. The most recognized are the bo, sai, nunchuaku, tonfa, and kama.

Unfortunately, due to sport karate's emphasis on aesthetic value, today many of the weapons true techniques are lost. They are usually replaced by flashy maneuvers used for winning contests. These endeavors usually bear little or no resemblance to good, effective Kobudo technique. Kobudo weapons are considered individual systems within a system so it is not uncommon to see them referred to in such a manner as bo-jutsu, sai-jutsu, or kama-jutsu. As mentioned earlier, the term jutsu means 'art,' so when one refers to bo-jutsu it literally means the 'art of the bo.'

Other less popular Kobudo systems include the *kama* or sickle, which was used to clear underbrush, the *kai*, or boat oar, whose techniques are based (in many cases) upon bojutsu methods, and the *suruchin*. The suruchin consists of a short length of rope or chain with weights on both ends that could be twirled in many ways and even thrown at the opponent. There was also *timbei*, a system which made use of a smaller, short-handled spear-like weapon. This was often used in concert with a straw hat, or a wooden or leather shield.

Of all the weapons in Kobudo, probably the most difficult to gain mastery of is the bo. Its techniques and principles can be considered

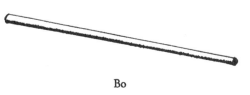

Bo

some of the most advanced within the Okinawan martial arts. Knowledge of basic empty-handed methods is somewhat helpful prior to undertaking study of the bo. The reason is that much of the footwork and stances used in bo-jutsu are very similar to that within the empty-handed methods. One common mistake made is equating Okinawan bo-jutsu with Japanese methods that involve the *yari* (spear) or naginata. These Japanese systems place greater emphasis upon the weapon itself and how much power can be generated from it. Traditionally, Chinese staffs and Okinawan bo differ in their physical characteristics. An Okinawan bo is tapered on its ends to help provide a stronger sense of focus when striking, whereas a Chinese staff is not.

The sai or short sword of Okinawan Kobudo can be found in a multitude of other Asian countries. Its presence on Okinawa is probably due to migrations from these regions. Many believe its point of origin to be Indonesia, a country with a long heritage of bladed fighting systems in its culture. In Okinawan Kobudo,

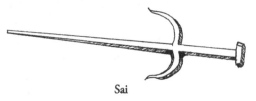

Sai

the sai has always been used in truncheon form and never as a bladed weapon. Sai techniques involve poking, stabbing, clubbing and even entrapping another weapon in its tines. The weapon is usually held in one of two positions. The first is with its shaft extended outward much the same way one would wield a sword or knife, the other position is with the shaft running the length of the practitioners forearm. Usually sai practitioners will alternate positions frequently depending upon the technique being executed. Normally three sai are carried. One for each hand and the third tucked into the belt. The third sai is most commonly used for throwing purposes. Supposedly an experienced sai practitioner can pin their opponents foot to the ground when throwing their sai.

Most Japanese fighting systems never officially accepted sai-jutsu into their ranks, although some may recently have adopted it. The majority of Japanese systems who do utilize sai-jutsu are usually of Okinawan ancestry, or else have been influenced by Okinawan Kobudo. Today it is still possible to see good sai-jutsu being practiced, but due to sport karate's influence, the majority of sai techniques are merely used as ornate extensions of the hands. Usually little attention is paid to proper execution of technique or sai-jutsu's role in Okinawan Kobudo.

Probably the most notable Kobudo weapon is the nunchuaku, which was made famous by the late Bruce Lee. The nunchuaku's original role was as an agricultural flail used in harvesting rice. Although considered secondary by some to other Kobudo systems, the nunchuakus development as a weapon is due mainly to Okinawan efforts. The nunchuaku can be used in a variety of ways, although it is most commonly used in a swinging or twirling method. The weapon can also be used for grappling and close quarters combat. Footwork involved in using the nunchuaku is very similar to Okinawan Karate or Te. Of all weapons, the nunchuaku are probably hardest to control during combat. If control over the weapon is lost, practitioners are just as likely to strike themselves as they are an opponent. It takes a skilled practitioner to strike with the nunchuaku and still maintain control over the weapon after its recoil. Like sai-jutsu, nunchuaku-jutsu today has lost much of its combat technique. In most cases combat techniques have been replaced by acrobatic twirling configurations which are designed for aesthetic grace and showmanship.

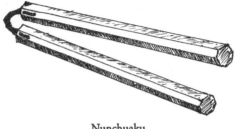

Nunchuaku

Tonfa-jutsu is another form of Kobudo whose development is due to Okinawan efforts. The tonfa was converted into a weapon due to Chinese influences and by applying principles utilized in sai-jutsu to it. Of all the Kobudo weapons applicable to empty-handed katas, the sai and tonfa are the two most readily available. Tonfa-jutsu techniques encompass many methods and include blocking, deflecting, entrapping, and elbowing to name just a few. The weapon is generally held in one of two fashions, the first being a reverse grip by the shaft using the handles as striking surfaces. The second is to hold the tonfa's handles with its shaft extending the length of ones forearm. The weapon can be used withdrawn with its shaft against the forearm, or in an extended position where it can be utilized like the nunchuaku in a swinging or twirling manner. The mark that distinguishes the expert from the novice is how well

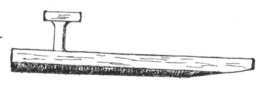

Tonfa

he can extend and retract the weapon from the forearm.

Today tonfa-jutsu is slowly disappearing from many karate schools. This is probably due to its lack of aesthetic value making it a somewhat unpopular weapon in tournament play. However, use of the tonfa has grown among many law enforcement agencies in recent years. The tonfa utilized by police officers is a somewhat modified version of the traditional weapon. It has a slightly longer shaft, and due to this additional length, it can also be employed as a riot baton, doubling the weapon's effectiveness.

One of the few bladed weapons of Okinawan Kobudo is the kama, which sometimes is mistaken for the Japanese kusarigama, a weapon used by the samurai. The kama is sickle-like tool used in cutting rice and can be found all throughout most of Asia. However, the Okinawans are given credit for utilizing this agricultural tool as an organized method of combat. The kusarigama has a somewhat larger blade than the kama. It also has a weighted chain attached to its handle that is used for ensnarling an opponents limbs. Although the two forms of fighting are considered different, there are similarities. Much of kama-jutsu's footwork is drawn from empty-handed methods of Te. In some instances however, the footwork has been modified to prevent the practitioners from injuring themselves with the weapon.

Kama

The kama can be utilized by holding the shaft with the weapon's blade pointing away from the practitioner, or with the shaft lying along the forearm and the blade pointed outward from the practitioner's elbows. This method of holding the kama is fairly common in close quarter combat. When held in this manner, the end of the kama's shaft can also be used for thrusting or poking type actions. As with the sai, nunchuaku, and tonfa, the kama can also be used for entrapping techniques.

Because it overlaps several empty-handed methods, in many cases, Kobudo makes up one-half of most Okinawan karate systems. Most systems of Okinawan karate have what is considered their own Kobudo kata. Often, these kata tend to be the favorites of a system's founder and are incorporated into their teachings. Isshin-ryu is one such system divided up this way, the Kobudo kata making up one-half of the sphere and empty-handed kata making up the other. Isshin-ryu utilizes Chatan Yara and Kusanku sai katas, Tokumine No Kon, Urasoe Bo, and Shushi No Kon Dai bo katas, the Chiefa tonfa kata, as well as Bo-To-Bo, and Bo-To-Sai pre-arranged kumite (sparring) forms. These forms make up Isshin-ryu's formation, however other Kobudo kata have been added depending upon the school or instructor's preference. This addition of Kobudo kata is also a common occurrence among other Okinawan systems of karate.

There are many reasons for including Kobudo kata within Okinawan karate. Some practitioner's state it was done to enhance empty-handed technique, others argue it was done for the preservation of Kobudo, another group says Kobudo was kept due to self-defense purposes. Something that cannot be denied is the Kobudo kata teach excellent armed methods of combat and practicing these forms will only enhance empty-handed techniques. Another somewhat overlooked point of interest concerning Kobudo, is that Kobudo kata can serve to remind us that the heritage of Okinawan systems are martial in nature. Because of the current popularity of sport karate, it might be easy to forget that.

In short, Kobudo's influence makes Okinawan karate a complete martial art. Kobudo's presence is well justified for without it, Isshin-ryu (or any other system of Okinawan karate for that matter) would not possess the depth or scope it holds today.

CHAPTER 3

Okinawan Karate—Its
Internal and External
Aspects

An old Chinese quote indicated that there are three categories of fighters. Type one recognizes only the hard aspects of boxing and relies entirely upon physical dexterity and quickness of eye. Type two recognizes only the internal aspects, believing that hard methods of training which stress physical dexterity are detrimental to the cultivation and flow of internal energy. Then there is the third category of fighter who recognizes both aspects of hard and soft and makes little distinction between them. Of these three categories, the third fighter is the most advanced.

Internal or 'soft' systems versus external or 'hard' forms of fighting. Which is superior? This is a very well worn argument in the martial arts community. For internal practitioners, the power behind their technique comes from the energy circulating in the body. *Chi*, a Chinese word, or *ki*, the Japanese variation, are terms used to describe the life force or internal energy believed to be within everyone. Practitioners of internal systems state that once mastered, use of chi is far more effective in overcoming an opponent than physical means. Many people find this concept hard to understand since some definitions of what chi actually is tend to border upon the mystical. Chi has many definitions and meanings. 'Spirit,' 'life force,' and 'natural energy' are just a few terms which have been used to describe this unseen phenomenon.

In contrast, external systems of fighting utilize quickness in eye and the body's muscular groups for power. Which is the superior method of practice? The answer is sort of like the, "which came first, the chicken or the egg" argument. Today the most widely recognized internal forms of martial arts are Aikido, Tai Chi, Hsing-I, and Pa Kua. Exponents of other systems such as karate, Shaolin boxing, or Tae Kwon Do will argue that chi can be developed even with heavy physical conditioning in training.

Traditionally, external systems are defined by the emphasis they place upon physical development and conditioning. For an external practitioner, their body must be capable of blocking and striking with tremendous force generated from the body's muscular and skeletal groups. Power for external techniques is generated from the practitioner's leg muscles used in a pushing or recoiling type of action. Power generated from this motion moves upward into the pelvic region where it is multiplied by rotation of the hips and upper body which transfers it through the striking arm. An external practitioner's muscular groups are trained to tense and relax at an instance. This is essential for quickness and developing maximum power in technique. External practitioners will also condition or toughen certain areas of their bodies. This is done to withstand blows or to inflict pain upon their opponent when blocking. In many instances, blocks used by hard systems are meeting force with force. The block's function is to stop an opponents strike and at the same time cause injury to the opponent. Such blocks are usually followed by powerful, thrusting hand or foot techniques.

Internal systems of fighting avoid training methods used by hard practitioners believing that they inhibit the flow of chi. For a soft practitioner calm mind, body structure, and continuity of motion are far more important than power or bold, aggressive actions. The legs of a soft stylist are expected to become powerful, yet their purpose is not for pushing or thrusting, but instead to provide a strong foundation for the practitioner's body. In practice, the internal practitioner's movements are usually executed slowly and very relaxed. The movements tend to be continuously flowing with little or no muscle power apparent during execution. Blocking and striking methods in internal systems are usually done in a soft, relaxed manner in circular motions. Blocking methods usually deflect oncoming blows and the blocking arm remains soft and relaxed, molding with the attack. Internal methods of blocking very seldom use force meeting force actions to stop a strike. An attack is deflected, redirected or avoided all together.

The geographical size of Okinawa facilitated a great deal of development between the various systems of fighting. Techniques, weapons, kata, and training methods for development of internal and external energy were all exchanged. Seldom will you find an absolutely hard or soft system of Okinawan karate. The emphasis on hard or soft technique within the system is usually left up to the individual instructor. Due to this constant blending of styles on Okinawa, Okinawan forms of karate at their more advanced levels can be described as middle forms, sort of a blend between internal and external. Not only do Okinawan practitioners utilize physical methods of conditioning, but soft principles are employed as well. For instance, many forms of blocking used in Isshin-ryu can be compared to the more circular motions of the softer Chinese styles.

Isshin-ryu karate, when first presented to the student, is basically taught as a linear system of fighting that utilizes hard blocking. This is a very simple yet effective way to start a beginning student's training. After a couple of years, angular movement and circular methods of blocking are brought to the student's attention. This development continues and relaxation and softness are stressed during the execution of technique. Soon the student is combining these elements with subtle shifting and slipping tactics, little movements that require little effort.

All of this development is based upon technique taught during the early stages of practice. In most cases with Isshin-ryu, there is little modification of technique needed. The system of Isshin-ryu however will change in some way for every practitioner over the course of time. The change may not be so much a physical change as much as a mental one. It could be argued that in many cases, one's mental outlook and how he chooses to approach his chosen art after years of study could be the distinguishing factor between its execution as an internal or external art.

The differences between the internal and external forms of Okinawan karate are at times vague. In defining the two, both certainly seem almost one in the same, especially in appearance. The contrast of body motion is not as apparent between hard and soft in Okinawan Karate as it might be between some Chinese systems.

Chang Sang Feng, who is credited with founding Tai Chi Chuan, once stated that the external systems differ in that they stress advancing and retreating, unison of hard and soft, and the conditioning or strengthening of muscle and bone. In contrast, internal systems place emphasis on defeating the opponent by placidness, the conditioning of bone and muscle, and overcoming one's opponent upon their initial attack. Both philosophies can be found in Okinawan karate, but separation of the two is still difficult at times. Perhaps with this in mind, we can erase some of the 'mystical' theories which are present and determine just which philosophy holds the greatest influence upon any given system of Okinawan karate.

One thing we may want to ask ourselves before labeling a system 'external' or 'internal' is to question more closely what chi really is and how we go about developing it. To date no one has bottled chi or for that matter presented physical evidence that this force exists. Many proclaim its existence, but just what exactly is it and how do proper body mechanics contribute to its development? One way to look at the development of chi is by first not attributing it to any one factor during training. It might be more helpful if we look at chi as something that is cultivated over a long period of time and results from the combination of all aspects of practice eventually 'coming together.' This 'coming together' is manifested when we see 60 and 70-year-old practitioners tossing opponents twice their size and half their age about the training hall effortlessly. Younger practitioners of the martial arts tend to rely heavily upon physical strength in execution of technique. This is because they have only a developing young body and their youthful strength to rely on.

On the other hand, older practitioners who have studied the martial arts for 40 or more years have a lifetime of practice to draw upon. Everything studied during their lifetime is executed naturally and with little or no thought given. It may be chi, it may be experience, or it could be both which makes these graying warriors such formidable opponents. The final decision is left to you.

CHAPTER 4

Religious Influences on Okinawan Karate

In recent years, due to television and movies, a great deal of reference has been made to the connection between the martial arts and religions such as Buddhism and Shintoism. Connections have even been drawn with other such philosophies like Zen or Taoism. Some of these connections and parallels being drawn are valid, while others are based purely upon romantic idealism.

Religious influences upon the martial arts can be traced back to when Bodhidharma, a Buddhist monk, journeyed from India to China. His original intentions upon arriving in China were to organize the various sects of Buddhism and to establish a monastery. After arriving however, Bodhidharma found Chinese monarchs did not accept his ideals. His original intentions left unfulfilled, Bodhidharma eventually gathered up a small group of followers and retreated into the wilderness. Once there, Bodhidharma and his followers constructed a temple known as the "Monastery of the Young Bamboo Forest," or Shaolin Temple as it is more popularly known. The temple would become the birthplace for Zen Buddhism and early Shaolin boxing methods.

Over time, Bodhidharma soon found his disciples weak from long hours of meditation and physical neglect. Bodhidharma himself was a skilled martial artist trained in an Indian fighting art known as Vajaramushti. To alleviate the monk's physical depletion Bodhidharma drew upon his own martial arts experience and devised a system of physical and mental exercises called I-Ching or 'inner conflicts.' This method of training would later come to be known as Sanchin in Okinawan karate. In addition, Bodhidharma also developed the 18 Hands of Lo Han, a system of unarmed combat used by the monks to protect themselves during their travels. Many of the philosophies of this fighting art were drawn directly from Buddhism. This is one of the earliest known influences of religion on the martial arts. From this beginning, Zen Buddhism and Shaolin fighting methods spread, sometimes hand in hand. Over the years other philosophies such as Taoism and Confucianism came to be incorporated into the martial arts. These philosophies were incorporated to instill a higher moral value in a system's practitioners. In other instances the philosophy was an inherent part of the system to begin with, much like the early Shaolin methods.

For instance, for the samurai warrior Zen Buddhism became a factor of day to day life that affected not only his personal affairs, but also the martial arts in which he trained. Zen Buddhism affected the samurai's virtues, teaching him that once a decision was reached, not to look back and to journey the course decided upon. In a philosophical sense, Zen taught the samurai to deal with matters of life and death with a very indifferent outlook. This state of mind allowed the samurai to remain undistracted by emotions, thoughts, or other matters that might affect his mental focus on the field of battle. This influence or incorporation of Buddhism into the samurai's art has also been carried over to many forms of Japanese martial arts today.

In dealing with Okinawan and Japanese martial arts one must keep in mind that both come from completely different cultural backgrounds. The differences however, may not be so apparent today as they were two hundred years ago. Today many people associate the two and their respective martial arts to be one and the same. This assumption has led many to believe that Okinawan karate is influenced by Buddhism or Zen. It is true that some of the Te techniques were brought to Okinawa by Buddhist monks, but while Okinawan arts were evolving, the fact remains that Buddhism was not a religion in great demand on Okinawa.

If one chooses to draw parallels between the Ryukyuan fighting arts and Buddhism, it is done without supporting evidence. It is important to note that Te began as a means of combat to be used against Japanese aggressors. Although the philosophy behind Okinawan karate has changed from that of a "martial art" to that of a "martial way," it was done so out of *philosophical* reasons and not *religious* ones. As for Japanese systems of karate, there is no evidence to be found in Funakoshi's original methods of teaching that suggests he was incorporating Buddhist aspects or Zen philosophies into his form of karate. Any such influence brought upon Japanese karate has been done so since the founding of Funakoshi's karate. It is human nature to romanticize, blow things out of proportion, or take them out of context. This holds especially true for many forms of Okinawan as well as Japanese karate. Much of the misunderstandings about the arts and comparisons and contrasts with various philosophies and religions have been brought forth by people such as writers or movie producers who have little or no experience in karate or the martial arts.

CHAPTER 5

The Introduction of Asian Fighting Arts and Isshin-Ryu to the United States

Asian fighting arts have been present in America for well over one hundred years. They found their way to this country through various means and methods—from service men who were stationed in Asia, from immigrants, and by members of large Asian corporations whose employees were assigned to work in the states.

The first people to bring Asian fighting arts into the United States were probably the Chinese immigrants brought to America during the 1850's to work on the Central Pacific railroad. Although many of these immigrants had knowledge of Chinese methods of boxing, it was kept within the Chinese communities and taught only amongst themselves. Most Okinawan and Japanese communities in the U.S. were also very secretive about their culture and martial art knowledge.

One of the earliest known public displays of any Asian fighting art to an American was in 1879 when President Grant visited Japan. While there, Grant observed a Judo demonstration at the Kodokan given by Jigoro Kano, the founder of Judo. Ten years later, Professor Ladd, an American scholar from Yale University, journeyed to Japan and began studying Judo at the Kodokan.

One of the first Asians to teach publicly in the United States was Yoshiaki Yamashita, a sixth dan in Kodokan Judo. While in the United States, Yamashita gave public demonstrations of Judo in New York and Chicago. During his stay in the U.S., Yamashita was invited to Washington D.C. to give a demonstration to President Theodore Roosevelt. Roosevelt was so impressed by Yamashita that he began studying Judo and went on to eventually earn a brown belt. Judo gained popularity in many American universities and eventually became the first Asian fighting art introduced to the American public on a grand scale. It would not be until after World War II however, when other Asian fighting arts like Okinawan and Japanese systems of karate, Burmese Bando, and internal and external methods of Chinese boxing would gain nationwide popularity.

One of the single greatest influences in the spread of Asian fighting arts to the United States was the return of American soldiers who were stationed abroad. Many of these men had been exposed to some form of Asian fighting art during their service. One of the first known karate dojos to be operated in the U.S. was by Robert Trias. Trias acquired his martial training while in the Navy. He taught a system of karate known as Shorei Goju-ryu and opened his school in 1946 in Phoenix, Arizona. Some of the other pioneers in U.S. martial arts were Anthony Mirikan (Goju-ryu), Cecil Patterson (Wado-ryu), Ed Parker (Kempo), Don Nagle and Steve Armstrong (Isshin-ryu), and George Mattson (Uechi-ryu.) The experiences of many of these early pioneers had varied from individual to individual. In some cases, practitioners spent up to twenty years in Asia under an instructor's tutelage, while other individuals received as little as a few months to a year of formal instruction.

The American military played both direct and indirect roles in the introduction of Asian fighting arts to the United States. As early as 1950, the Air Force began setting up Judo programs for its aircrews to learn hand-to-hand combat. Later, the Air Force would send personnel to Japan to train in both Judo and Shotokan karate. Many of those sent ended up studying under some of Funakoshi's more well known students like Masatoshi Nakayama, Isao Obata, and Hidetake Nishiyama. After their return to the U.S., these airmen began teaching combat air crews hand-to-hand tactics as well as opening karate and judo clubs on Air Force bases. After their discharge from the Air Force, some would begin teaching karate and judo in the civilian sectors.

The Air Force was not the only branch of armed forces to institute hand-to-hand combat programs. The Army, Navy, and Marine Corps all had similar programs. Aside from the daily hand-to-hand training, the military also promoted practice of the martial arts among its members stationed in Asia. As the story goes, in the early 1950's the Marines would pay five dollars a month per marine to one of the local Okinawans for karate lessons. As it turned out, that certain Okinawan happened to be Tatsuo Shimabuku and his system was called Isshin-ryu.

Tatsuo Shimabuku allegedly gained the attention of Marines stationed on Okinawa during a karate demonstration. Shimabuku was attempting to drive a nail into a board with his fist and for some reason, he missed the nail and cut his hand. Shimabuku simply picked up a handful of dirt, placed it on the wound and continued on with the demonstration. Afterwards some of the Marines present sought Shimabuku out for instruction and helped him secure a teaching position with the Marines. It would be these Marines and the ones who followed that would be instrumental in introducing Isshin-ryu karate to the United States. Probably four of the most well known individuals to start studying under Tatsuo Shimabuku during the early 1950's are Harold Mitchum, Don Nagle, Steve Armstrong, and Harold Long. Around this time, Shimabuku officially formed the Isshin-ryu system.

Harold Mitchum was a career Marine and began practicing with Shimabuku in 1954. Mitchum ended up spending seven and a half years on Okinawa studying under Shimabuku. In addition to Isshin-ryu, Mitchum also studied Shorin-ryu karate. In 1961 Mitchum was appointed by Shimabuku to be the first president of the American Okinawan Karate Association. Currently Mitchum is retired from the Marines and heads up the United Isshin-ryu Karate Association in Albany, Georgia.

Don Nagle was the first Marine to return from Okinawa and open up an Isshin-ryu dojo in the United States. Nagle began his study of Isshin-ryu in 1955 and, while still a white belt, won the Okinawa Karate Championships. Nagle returned to the United States in 1957 and opened his first dojo in Jacksonville, North Carolina. Nagle is noted for being one of first people to bring Isshin-ryu to the United States and for opening one of the first karate dojos in the southeastern

United States. After his discharge from the Marines, Nagle moved to New Jersey, where he opened a second dojo. Nagle passed away in 1999.

Prior to his study of Isshin-ryu, Steve Armstrong had studied Goju-ryu and Shorin-ryu while stationed in Japan, earning second degree black belts *(ni-dans)* in both systems. In addition, before joining the Marines, Armstrong was also an amateur boxer, wining 68 out of 72 bouts. This boxer turned karate-ka served in Korea and later in Washington, D.C. Armstrong began studying Isshin-ryu in 1956. When he told Shimabuku

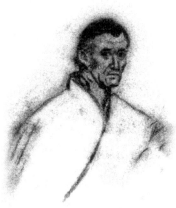

Don Nagle

that he already held two ni-dan rankings, Shimabuku reportedly laughed at him and would only permit him to wear a white belt during his workouts. Only after four or five months would Shimabuku allow Armstrong to wear a black belt.

Armstrong returned from Okinawa around 1960 and eventually opened his own Isshin-ryu school in Tacoma, Washington. Shimabuku considered Armstrong second in command to Harold Mitchum in the American Okinawan Karate Association. Armstrong later became president of the association. After many years as its director, he turned over control of the organization to Lou Lizotte, another one of Shimabuku's early students.

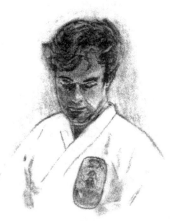

Steve Armstrong

Harold Long began his studies under Shimabuku in 1956. Long allegedly studied as long as eight hours a day, seven days a week during his 17 month stay on Okinawa. After he was discharged from the Marines, Long returned to Knoxville Tennessee in 1959 and started teaching soon thereafter. In 1974 Long returned to Okinawa to confer with Tatsuo Shimabuku about founding the International Isshin-ryu Karate Association. He was elected as the organization's first president with its board of directors being Harry Acklin, Ed Johnson, and Harold Mitchum. He has also co-authored a series of books with Allen Wheeler, founder of the Okinawan Karate-Do Union, titled *Dynamics of Isshin-ryu Karate*. After a very distinguished history in the martial arts, Long died in 1998.

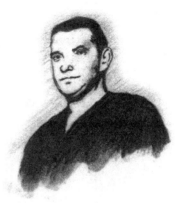

Harold Long

The individuals mentioned above contributed greatly to the spreading of Isshin-ryu throughout the United States. They are some of the best known because they are the Isshin-ryu pioneers. They were either the first to open Isshin-ryu dojos in the states or they eventually became leaders of Isshin-ryu organizations in the United States. These four were not the only people to study under Shimabuku, however. There were many others who spent time on Okinawa under Shimabuku's instruction. The following are some of those less recognized karate-ka.

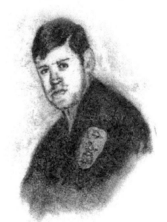

William Gardo

William Gardo began studying the martial arts in 1958. It was not until 1961 that he began his study under Tatsuo Shimabuku. Gardo trained for two and a half years with Shimabuku. While on Okinawa, he also studied Goju-ryu, Shorin-ryu, Uechi-ryu, Pa Kua, and Okinawan Kobudo. Gardo returned to the United States in 1964 and later organized the Dixie National Karate Association.

Tom Lewis was stationed on Okinawa with the Marine Corps in 1959. That same year he began studying Isshin-ryu. Lewis was on Okinawa for 18 months. Aside from studying with Tatsuo Shimabuku, he also worked out with Don Nagle, Steve Armstrong, Harold Michum, Rick Niemera and Donald Bohan. Lewis is also a member of the American Bando Association and the author of *Karate For Kids*.

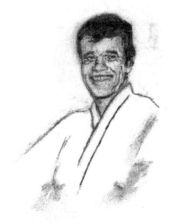

Tom Lewis

Jim Advincula was a career Marine who began his study of Isshin-ryu in the 1950's. Advincula spent seven to ten years on Okinawa under Shimabuku's instruction. Jim is a multi-talented martial artist studying not only Okinawan Karate and Kobudo, but other systems such as Philippine Escrima and Judo. Advincula currently resides in San Diego, California, where he operates his own Isshin-ryu dojo. He has also been featured in *Black Belt* magazine.

John Bartosivich is probably one of the most knowledgeable of the Isshin-ryu pioneers, but also one of the least recognized nationally. A career Marine, John spent close to 14 years on and off Okinawa studying Isshin-ryu— most of it under Shimabuku's guidance. Bartosivitch has been

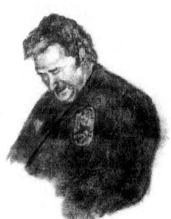

Rick Niemera

called one of the top fighters and Kobudo practitioners in the Isshin-ryu system.

Rick Niemera began his study of karate in the early 1950's under Shimabuku. Not only did Niemera study Isshin-ryu, but he also practiced Bando with Muang Gyi and ended up attaining high ranking in both systems. Niemera was very proficient in Isshin-ryu, Bando, and their related weapons systems. He was also recognized as being an outstanding fighter and an excellent street tactician.

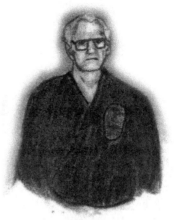
Don Bohan

Don Bohan was another respected Isshin-ryu pioneer who, along with spending a good number of years on Okinawa studying with Shimabuku, also practiced with Don Nagle. Bohan was noted for his expertise in the practical applications of kata *(bunkai)* and possessed a very great understanding of the historical aspects of Asian martial arts. Bohan was affiliated with the American Bando Association and died in 1998.

Sherman Harrell is still yet another Marine who studied with Shimabuku in the late 1950's and early 1960's. Unlike many others, Harrell did not start teaching publicly when he returned to the states. Harrell kept somewhat of a low profile until around 1985, when he became affiliated with the Okinawan Karate-Do Union. Harrell is known not as a specialist in any one field, but instead as a solid, all-around practitioner. One of Harrell's sayings is that he's had two instructors in his lifetime—Tatsuo Shimabuku and the Isshin-ryu kata.

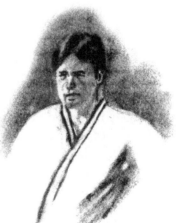
Sherman Harrell

These are only a few of the earliest Isshin-ryu pioneers. Some were able to start teaching almost immediately after returning to the U.S., making their impact felt almost instantly in the civilian sector and capitalizing off the growing interest in the martial arts. Others, like the career Marines, were not able to do so due to the nature of the military. They were however, able to teach classes on military installations or in the surrounding communities. One advantage these men had was their ability to stay longer on Okinawa and continue their own training.

Discussing these early Isshin-ryu pioneers brings to light a curious habit Shimabuku had when many of the Marines left Okinawa. Shimabuku would usually promote a departing Marine to a high rank, possibly as high as fifth or sixth dan. This caused quite a commotion because many of the Marines Shimabuku promoted had barely two years of study. To obtain such a rank under normal circumstances would usually require 13 or more years. Many have questioned this act and asked if these Marines were really that proficient after only two years or less. The answer is that they were not—*at that point in time.* Today however, many of these men have over 30 years in Isshin-ryu and now quite deserving of their rank.

Harold Mitchum once said that Shimabuku knew what he was doing regarding the premature promotions he bestowed on departing Marines.

Shimabuku apparently was well aware that students who have only been studying for one year did not deserve such a rank, but he also realized that it was more than likely he would never see many of these men again. For them to be able to effectively spread Isshin-ryu throughout the United States and to establish and lead its various organizations, they would need to have the credentials to do so. These promotions were, in effect, credentials

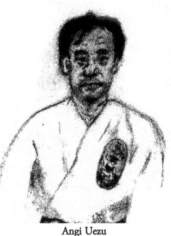

Angi Uezu

that would allow these men to carry out the task of introducing Isshin-ryu to the United States.

Although not American karate pioneers, two other practitioners should be mentioned. They are Kichiro Shimabuku,

Tatsuo Shimabuku's son and current head of the Isshin-ryu
World Karate Association and Angi Uezu, Tatsuo's son-in-law.
Both men have played significant roles in Isshin-ryu's later day
developments. Like many of the soldiers, Angi and Kichirio
began studying with Shimabuku during the late 1950's or
early 1960's. It is interesting to note that these two influential
figures are junior to some of the Marines who began prior to
Angi and Kichrio—a fact which caused some controversy as to
who would lead Isshin-ryu after Shimabuku's death.

Political Organizations. Within Isshin-ryu today there are
five major political organizations and many minor ones. The
major organizations are:

- Isshin-ryu World Karate Association founded by
  Kichiro Shimabuku.
- International Isshin-ryu Karate Association founded
  by Harold Long.
- Okinawan Karate-Do Union founded by Allen
  Wheeler.
- United Isshin-ryu Karate Association by Harold
  Mitchum.
- American Okinawan Karate Association formed by
  Shimabuku, Harold Mitchum, and Steve Armstrong.
- Professional Isshin-ryu Karate Federation founded by
  Joseph Jennings.
- United States Isshinryu Karate Association, founded
  by Phil Little, with the blessing of Harold G. Long.

Allen Wheeler was not one of the original Marines to
study with Shimabuku nor was Joseph Jennings. Wheeler was
a long time student of Harold Long before founding the
Okinawan Karate-Do Union, and Jennings' organization has
ties with Angi Uezu. The organizations within Isshin-ryu have
helped it to become one of the fastest growing and most popular systems of karate today, They have however, also brought
much turmoil due to competition and political infighting
among organizations and members.

After returning to America, some of the original pioneers
of Isshin-ryu found it difficult to preserve the system as it had
been taught to them. Movements of the kata were lost or

changed due to human error. More importantly, Shimabuku had taught some of his pupils slightly different variations of the kata than he had others. After some of the earlier pioneers had left Okinawa, Shimabuku continued to experiment and even alter the kata. According to Angi Uezu, this is one reason why many later day students' kata differs from those of the earlier students.

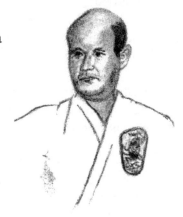

In 1966, Shimabuku journeyed to America. While he was here, a film was made of him performing empty-handed and Kobudo katas. This was done in an attempt to maintain uniformity in the teaching of these forms. Some organizations use this film as the final word on Shimabuku's teachings, while others interpret it a bit more liberally.

Kichiro Shimabuku

These factors, along with people's egos, have done much to promote disharmony within Isshin-ryu. However, if you look at the differences in kata (usually one of the biggest sources of tension between organizations) it is more than likely that the differences are in the kata's *technique* and not its *principles*. More often than not, the kata are actually quite similar.

Changing kata for "change's sake" is not necessarily the best way to maintain the principles being taught by the form. However, when change is made for the better, *by people with the experience to make such changes,* the form evolves for the better—a principle that Shimabuku himself would no doubt agree.

CHAPTER 6

Shuri-Te and Naha-Te Influences on Isshin-Ryu

Frequently the term Shuri-te is used generically to refer to Shorin-ryu or any other form of karate from Shuri. Likewise, Naha-te tends to be used when referring to Goju-ryu and Uechi-ryu. This is a common practice among Okinawan karate-ka when speaking of their system's lineage. Isshin-ryu karate is an eclectic system, meaning that Shimabuku combined what he considered to be the best aspects of Goju-ryu and Shorin-ryu into his form of karate. When a system is founded, it is by an individual who is utilizing aspects that best express his own interpretation and understanding of the martial arts. Shimabuku borrowed from Shorin-ryu and Goju-ryu what he *felt were the most appropriate techniques, tactics, and principles to express his interpretation of Okinawan karate.*

Isshin-ryu practitioners are fond of saying that the art is drawn from Shorin-ryu and Goju-ryu. It might be true that Isshin-ryu's immediate influences are drawn from these two systems, but to end the debate here would not do justice to the art or its founder.

As mentioned earlier, because Okinawa was so small, there was a great deal of influence between the arts. It would be hard, if not impossible, to find an art that completely stood alone and remained untouched by any other arts of the day. Isshin-ryu's influences, like most other Okinawan systems, can be traced back to the earliest days in Ryukyuan history when empty-handed forms of fighting were simply known as Te. Going further back, we would be able to find a line leading back to the original Shaolin temple when Sanchin principles were taught to monks by Bodhidarama. Today however, most people speak in terms of more immediate influences on Okinawan karate, with Isshin-ryu practitioners categorizing them into three groups—Kobudo, Shorin-ryu, and Goju-ryu. Shimabuku was a noted practitioner of all three of these groups.

Shobayashi Shorin-ryu, first taught by Chotoku Kyan, is the source of the major Shuri-te influences on Isshin-ryu. The Seisan, Naihanchi, Wansu, Chinto, and Kusanku katas are taken from the Shobaysahi-ryu. Shimabuku did not use the Pinan katas, which many Shorin-ryu schools utilize. Shuri-te systems and later Shorin-ryu forms of Okinawan karate were strongly influenced by external methods of Chinese boxing. In turn Shuri-te, along with systems that evolved from it, tend to be somewhat more physical and offensive than those of Naha-te.

Shuri-te or Shorin-ryu tends to rely upon upright stances, and encompasses linear and angular types of body movement with quick movements to the front and rear. Although most blocking and parrying in Okinawan karate is circular in nature, Shuri-te systems do employ some hard blocking methods. To pick out these influences in Isshin-ryu, all one has to do is observe the Kusanku or Chinto katas. Their body movements are as described above—light and rapid from shallow stances with quick movement to one's front and rear. Hard blocking methods are not utilized in Isshin-ryu as they sometimes are in Shorin-ryu.

Shallow stances are very apparent in Shimabuku's karate. Watching an Isshin-ryu practitioner perform kata will certainly confirm this. However, it is felt that the shallow stances in Isshin-ryu come not only from Shuri-te, but from Naha-te as well. By omitting long, lunging-type movements, Shimabuku allows for more footwork and body movement. Freedom from deeper stances allow the practitioner to perform subtle slipping, weaving, and bobbing movements. Such actions require agile footwork that can be greatly restricted when performed from deeper stances. The soft blocking, in conjunction with the Shorin-ryu kata, shallow stances, and lack of lunging-type movements help to greatly distinguish Isshin-ryu from other systems of Okinawan karate.

In some ways the Shorin-ryu kata can be considered the foundation from which Isshin-ryu is built. However, Isshin-ryu not only uses Shorin-ryu's methods of movement, but those of Naha-te as well, giving it not only angular and linear, but also semicircular body movements. Naha-te, and the systems that evolved out of it, fell primarily under the influence of internal methods. Shimabuku was a noted Goju-ryu practitioner, having studied under Chojun Miyagi, the founder. The word Goju is composed of two characters. 'Go' meaning 'hard,' and "Ju" which denotes 'soft,' 'pliable,' or 'gentle.' The name greatly reflects upon the system that contains both hard and soft methods. Roughly 75% of the techniques in Goju-ryu are done with the hands. The remaining 15% are executed with the feet. Isshin-ryu also divides its techniques roughly along these same lines. Many of Isshin-ryu's grappling, throwing, and entrapping techniques come from Goju-ryu along with the emphasis placed on medium to close-quarters fighting, something Isshin-ryu is also noted for.

Isshin-ryu inherits both the Seiuchin and Sanchin katas from Goju-ryu. There are two stories behind the origins of this form. One claims that Chojun Miyagi devised the kata, and the other says that its roots can be traced back to the Chinese internal methods of Hsing-I or Pa Kua. Seiuchin is noted for its graceful flowing movements, many of which can be used in grappling applications. Most of the kata is performed from a horse-riding stance, and it is quite unique in that there is not a single kicking technique in the entire form.

The Sanchin kata has been described as the backbone of Isshin-ryu karate. If you point out any one single Goju influence that has contributed the most to Isshin-ryu, it would probably be Sanchin. This form's history can be traced back to the original Shaolin temple when Bodhidarama introduced Sanchin-type exercises to the monks as a form of physical and mental conditioning. Sanchin's early evolution is due to Zen Buddhism, and although Okinawan karate as a whole was not heavily influenced by religion, some aspects of Zen Buddhism are present today due to the Sanchin kata. One of the many aspects stressed in Sanchin practice is the concept of standing or moving Zen—a philosophy rooted in Zen Buddhism used to help the practitioner achieve total enlightenment.

Very simply put, Zen can be summed up as a state of 'no mind' in which the everyday processes of thinking is set aside.

One attempts to uncloud the mind, allow it to relax, and focuses entirely upon the task at hand with little regard given to one's success or failure, life or death. The only mindset is one of 'there only is.' Standing or moving Zen encompasses the same concepts except mental and physical elements of the practitioner are functioning as a whole. Sanchin is a powerful form and contributes both mentally and physically to the practitioner. Along with helping to coordinate mind and body, Sanchin is very effective in developing the muscular, cardiovascular, and skeletal systems. Sanchin practice also develops dynamic tension, proper breathing and bone strength, all of which are essential qualities for an effective fighter.

Up until now, we've covered some aspects that Isshin-ryu utilized from other systems of Okinawan karate, but what about the concepts that were not adopted into Isshin-ryu? What effect does their absence have on Shimabuku's karate? Two things most practitioners from other systems note about Isshin-ryu is that there are no kicking techniques above the solar plexus and that the footwork lacks deep forward and back stances. These are very common in many forms of Japanese karate. Postures like the *zenkutsu dachi* (forward stance) or *kokutsu dachi* (back stance) are widely used in Shotokan and Wado-ryu. Deep frontal or backward leaning-type stances are used in almost every system of karate or Chinese boxing currently practiced. In many cases, a practitioner sacrifices mobility for power by utilizing such postures. The advantage of using deep stances however, is that that it helps beginning students develop excellent leg muscles and allows them to achieve a lower center of gravity. Shallow methods of footwork are used in Isshin-ryu with the only deep stance being the 'horse riding' stance.

Some forms of Okinawan karate like Goju-ryu utilize high kicking techniques along with exaggerated stances. The purpose is not so much of a combative nature as it is one of physical development. Practicing deep stances and high kicking promotes a strong sense of balance, flexibility, endurance, and strength in the practitioner's legs. However, the practicality of using high-kicking techniques in a close-quarter combative situation is very debatable. Isshin-ryu's kicking techniques are unique in that they are all based on a snapping or whipping type actions. All kicks travel a direct course to their target. There are no spinning kicks, and most of the foot techniques can be used in close-quarter situations. Isshin-ryu's foot strikes are very combative in nature and reflect back to the kicking methods of early Te systems.

There are pros and cons to the exclusion of other traditional methods of training when looking at Isshin-ryu. It should be noted that one of the underlying principles behind Shimabuku's system is that there are few big movements. It is a system of fighting based on direct reaction to an opponents attack. This is one reason stances such as *zenkutsu dachi* were omitted by Shimabuku. Their performance does not facilitate the type of movement utilized in Isshin-ryu. Rather than have a new student begin a system of karate whose initial teachings are more oriented towards physical development than combative effectiveness, the Isshin-ryu practitioner instead begins in a system combative in nature. Because some of the techniques learned in Isshin-ryu are almost instantly applicable, one may question the benefits of beginning at the so-called 'end.' Some system's techniques will physically change in execution and appearance over the years. In many cases, the novice begins with big, force-on-force type, linear movements. After years of study however, his movements become very small, soft, and subtle.

Isshin-ryu techniques need little, if any refining. The disadvantage however, is that from day one, the Isshin-ryu practitioner is practicing a refined product. The student has not seen the technique develop from infancy to its current stages, and therefore has no standard of comparison. They cannot compare the technique as it was taught from beginning, to intermediate, to advanced levels. This leads to many misconceptions about the nature of Isshin-ryu. Some of the best Isshin-ryu practitioners are individuals who have studied other systems of karate prior to taking up Shimabuku's art. These individuals already had a great deal of experience to fall back on and had a set standard of comparison. I once heard Isshin-ryu karate described by another practitioner as, "one of those systems where you spend thirty years practicing a martial art and then take up the study of Isshin-ryu."

Although one of the many redeeming qualities of Isshin-ryu is its simplicity, many of the misconceptions drawn about the system come from its own practitioners. Some will describe Shimabuku's karate as a linear system of fighting that utilizes hard blocking. Others will place great emphasis on hand and foot technique, but pay little or no attention to principles of body movement and postures. Simply observing the footwork of the art will make one realize that it is not a hard system. The shallow seisan stance is the workhouse of the system's footwork. The smaller, narrow, circular stepping that normally accompanies seisan is simply not designed to support hard force-meeting-force type actions. Three of the underlying principles in Isshin-ryu are simplicity, subtleness, and effectiveness. When one compares an Isshin-ryu kata to a Shorin-ryu form for example, these principles are easily defined. The Isshin-ryu kata have been influenced by Shorin-ryu Goju-ryu, Kobudo, and Shimabuku's own innovations. It has been said that if it came down to tradition or effectiveness, Shimabuku was a man known to choose the latter. He was known for his innovations in the karate world.

One of Shimabuku's innovations with the Isshin-ryu kata is that all techniques are performed in a manner very similar to the way they would be utilized in combat. None of the movements are performed for aesthetic value or to hide certain techniques of the form, a practice sometimes found in other systems of karate. Isshin-ryu is also one of the first systems of Okinawan karate in the latter 20th century to omit the use of Pinan katas. Instead, the beginning student learns the more advanced Dan katas. In place of Pinan, Shimabuku devised a series of blocking and striking combinations known as "the charts." These basic blocks and strikes encompass many of the basic methods of movement and body postures found throughout Isshin-ryu. By practicing the charts, the Isshin-ryu practitioner is able to break down the system into its most minute form of study.

In recent years however, some schools of Isshin-ryu have started teaching either Shorin-ryu or Goju-ryu Pinan kata. One reason for this is that some people feel that starting a beginning student on advanced forms is too difficult. Some other schools have even devised their own Isshin-ryu forms. We have already seen that it is extremely difficult to attempt to classify Ryukyuan arts as hard or soft, and Isshin-ryu is no exception. It is not uncommon to find some dojos stressing either a hard or soft form in their teachings, while others will teach Isshin-ryu as a middle system with influences bordering on both.

Recently there have been attempts to link Isshin-ryu to various forms of Japanese karate, specifically Shotokan. While it is true that Shimabuku was a very innovative man who would borrow anything if he felt it was useful, there is no evidence to suggest that he took techniques from Shotokan. Some of the inherent similarities between Isshin-ryu and Shotokan are due to the fact that both are direct descendants of Shuri-te systems of fighting, and both have a good deal of the same kata and techniques. However, if one wishes to examine any other influences (outside of Ryukyuan fighting arts) found in Isshin-ryu, it would be wise to look towards China, as this is where most Okinawans journeyed when they wished to further expand their knowledge of the martial arts.

CHAPTER 7

Tatsuo Shimabuku—Isshin-Ryu's Founder and His Instructors

We've looked at the systems that have contributed to Isshin-ryu, now we will examine the people who helped in its founding. Personalities play a major role in the practice of a martial art, for it is the individual and their own likes and dislikes which ultimately determine what kind of system is to be practiced. Two Isshin-ryu stylists for example may practice the same system, but their karate will differ due to each individuals body size, agility, preference in technique, and even interpretation of techniques within kata (*bunkai*).

This "personality factor" plays an even larger role in the development of a fighting system. Shimabuku has been described by many as a very practical and realistic man. These traits carried over into Isshin-ryu as philosophies of no wasted movement, and responding directly to an assailant's attack. Before examining Tatsuo Shimabaku and his instructors, let us discuss one other factor. Much has been made today about one's "founding" a martial system. While many agree it is beneficial to pursue other arts, others disagree with breaking away from the teachings of a traditional system and one's instructor.

It is important to note that the "founding" of a martial art was a very common occurrence not just in the Ryukyu islands, but in Japan, China, Korea, and Europe as well. Had certain individuals decided not to break off, we would not have such systems as Aikido, Judo, Wado-ryu, Shotokan Tae Kwon Do, and a host of others. The formalization and teaching of an individual's personal interpretation of the martial arts is a natural occurrence. It is the result of years of practice and takes place at an extremely high level of development, even if no formal name is adopted or no ties are broken with one's teacher.

Today many American martial artists will point to the Okinawans and say, "They did it, so why can't I?" It is extremely important to note that Tatsuo Shimabuku had over 44 years of experience in the martial arts when he officially founded Isshin-ryu karate. Today it is fairly common to find Americans with this much time spent studying the martial arts whose experience, like Shimabuku's, is based on good, sound technique and principles learned from qualified instructors. As the martial arts become more deeply ingrained in American society, we will find more and more of these very qualified individuals founding their own systems. These truly talented individuals are quite a find indeed, and very much the exception rather than the rule. Nowadays we see the foundation of many systems of American karate by individuals with very little formal instruction in the martial arts—practitioners whose experience is based on tournament play and not true martial principles or techniques.

The world has become a lot smaller with, among other things, the advent of trains, planes, automobiles, and computers. These innovations have had a tremendous impact on the martial arts. Today the arts are widespread, but in Shimabuku's day, the Ryukyuan martial arts community was close knit with a rather structured hierarchy. This governing body, along with the social and cultural values of the day, helped prevent the founding of systems with little or no martial value to them. His was also an era before sport karate, a time in which the practice and understanding of sound technique determined who might live or die, not who would receive a championship trophy. Tatsuo Shimabuku's instructors were all of this era. Most were born and began practicing the Ryukyuan-te systems when there was a great deal of secrecy surrounding them. This secrecy was due to Japanese laws forbidding practice of any martial art by the Okinawans.

The four most widely recognized of Tatsuo Shimabuku's instructors are Chotoku Kyan, Choki Motobu, Chojun Miyagi, and Taira Shinken. Although one can assume Shimabuku trained with many other notable instructors, these four individuals are widely recognized as his formal instructors who contributed the most to his martial development. There are other instructors however, that also contributed to

Shimabuku's growth along the way. They are Irshu Matsumora (Shuri-te), Yabiku Moden (Okinawan Kobudo), and Gajoko Chioyu (Shimabuku's uncle and a noted Shuri-te master.) It was Gajoko Chioyu who first introduced a young Shimabuku to Chotoku Kyan.

Kyan was born in 1870 in Shuri. He was a slim man who, as a youth, led a rather sickly childhood. His father, a proficient Shuri-te practitioner in his own right, gave Kyan some of his first lessons in Sumo and Okinawan Te. As Kyan's interests and abilities grew, his father realized that he could not impose the severity upon his son needed to bring forth his true abilities. It was at this time when he asked Matsumora Kosaku, a noted Tomari-te master, to teach his son. Kyan eventually became very proficient in Tomari-te and later began the study of Shuri-te under the instruction of Bushi Matsumura. Allegedly, the training Matsumura imposed on Kyan was much more severe than anything he could have been subjected to in a Zen temple.

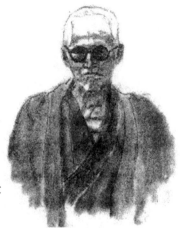

Chotoku Kyan

It was Matsumura who taught the Chinto and Seisan katas to Kyan, both of which Matsumura learned from Sakugawa, another Okinawan karate great. Kyan was noted for his mastery of ki, his extremely proficient foot techniques, and for practicing Seisan diligently. Before the introduction of karate into the Okinawan school system in 1903, Seisan was traditionally the first kata taught. However, when karate was first introduced into schools, Pinan forms replaced Seisan as the first form. Kyan never made the switch over however, and continued the tradition of teaching Seisan first—a trait later adopted by Tatsuo Shimabuku in Isshin-ryu. Kyan never considered himself a specialist, and was well versed in all aspects of the arts. He later went on to form the Shobayashi-ryu system of Shorin-ryu karate, the leadership of which was passed to Eizo Shimabuku, Tatsuo's younger brother and also a student of Kyan.

"The body of a bull and the spirit of a saint" is a phrase commonly used to describe Chojun Miyagi. Miyagi was born to an wealthy family in 1888. Because he really didn't have to worry about money, he was able to devote his life to the study of karate. Miyagi began his study of Naha-te at the early age of nine under the guiding hand of Kanryu Higashionna, who is commonly recognized as the father of Naha-te. Higashionna studied internal systems of boxing for close to 20 years while he was in China. Until this point, the Ryukyuan fighting arts (with a few exceptions) had been practiced in more of an external fashion. Higashionna's return to Okinawa brought about a stronger influence of the internal aspects. Miyagi studied with Higashionna until his death in 1915. After his teacher's death, Miyagi ventured to China on two separate occasions where he studied both internal and external methods of Chinese boxing, one of which was Pa Kua. He later organized this knowledge and his mastery of Naha-te into a system now known as Goju-ryu style.

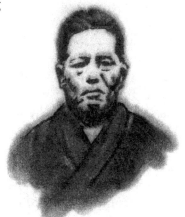

Chojun Miyagi

Miyagi went to great lengths to internationalize Okinawan karate. He traveled to Japan and Hawaii, and he also gave demonstrations of his Goju system. In 1933, Miyagi went before the Dai Nippon Budo Kai that, at the time, was the largest Japanese martial arts federation recognized by the Japanese government. Miyagi, representing the Okinawan martial arts, gave a presentation called, "An Outline of Karate-Do." Like Funakoshi, Miyagi's presentation enabled some systems of karate being practiced in Japan to be recognized as "official" Japanese martial arts. This presentation also resulted in Miyagi's being awarded the title of master, the first such title to be officially awarded by the Dai Nippon Budo Kai. In 1935 he was awarded a professor's degree from the organization. Later that year, Miyagi returned to Okinawa.

Besides Tatsuo Shimabuku, Miyagi also taught other famous martial artists, one of which was Gogen Yamaguchi, commonly referred to by his nickname, "The Cat." Yamaguchi began studying karate under Miyagi around 1929, and in 1935 he organized the All Japan Goju Kai Karate-Do Association. Miyagi died in 1953 and was succeeded by Meitoku Yagi, a long time student and a man who is considered to be world's foremost authority on Goju karate today.

One of Shimabuku's more colorful instructors was Choki Motobu. Motobu was born to nobility in 1871 and was one of three sons. His father, Chomura, was a grandmaster of a fighting system taught only to members of Motobu's family. The system was known as Motobu-ryu and in many ways held strong resemblance to Aiki-jutsu. The elder Motobu passed on his teaching to the family's oldest son Choyu, who then refused to instruct Choki in the system because of his character.

Choki set out to learn karate on his own. He often practiced by himself by punching on the makiwara board and lifting heavy stones to develop his strength. Motobu developed his own fighting techniques and strategies and then went into Shuri, where he would instigate fights to see if his combative theories were valid. Some considered Motobu more of a brawler than a martial artist. He was reportedly a man more at

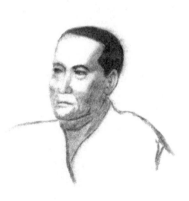

Choki Motobu

home in the mist of a street fight than a dojo. Because of his reputation, many Okinawan karate masters refused to teach him. Some had even fallen prey to Motobu's abilities, which further increased the feelings of animosity towards him.

One of Miyagi's first instructors was Kosaku Matsumora, a Tomari-te master. Matsumora eventually took on Motobu as a student because he was impressed by his determination and ability. Matsumora taught Motobu kata hoping it would calm his aggressive nature. He refused, however, to teach sparring technique. Motobu, not easily dissuaded, would sneak in and watch Matsumora training with other students. Eventually, Motobu learned the Naihanchi and Passai katas from Matsumora.

Motobu moved to Osaka, Japan in 1921. During that year at a public exhibition, Motobu gained national fame by knocking out the European heavyweight boxing champ. Motobu lived in Japan for close to 15 years, during which time he opened a dojo in Tokyo. In 1936, Motobu returned to Okinawa to further his knowledge of Okinawan karate and Kobudo. Upon his return, he studied under Kentsu Yabu, one of only a handful of men ever to defeat him in a match. During his later years, Motobu began to study karate for more spiritual purposes and placed more emphasis on kata than kumite. Motobu died in 1944 and his teachings are carried on by one of his more notable students—Shoshin Nagamine, leader of Matsubayshi Shorin-ryu.

Taira Shinken was born on the tiny island of Kume. He studied Kobudo under Moden Yabiku. Shinken also studied karate under such greats as Yasutsune Azato, Yasutsune Itosu, and Kentsu Yabu. Shinken traveled frequently to Japan staying sometimes for as long as six to eight months. During these visits Shinken also studied karate with Gichin Funakoshi. Shinken was not Shimabuku's first Kobudo instructor, (Shimabuku received instructed in Kobudo from Chotoku Kyan). Shinken, however, is the one history credits with having the most influence in Shimabuku's Kobudo training. He has also been called one of the greatest Kobudo masters in Okinawan history. In 1935, he founded the Society for

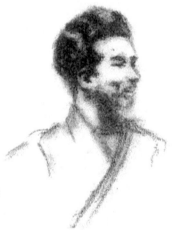

Taira Shinken

Preservation and Promotion of Ryukyuan Martial Arts. Many karate greats studied with Shinken—Eizo Shimabuku, Tatsuo

Shimabuku, Fumio Demura, Ryusho Sakagami, and Motokatsu Inoue among others. Upon his death in 1970, Inoue succeeded Shinken as the leader of the Ryukyuan Martial Arts Society.

Shimabuku—The Man. Tatsuo Shimabuku was born at the turn of the century around 1906 or 1908. His original name was Shinkichi, but he later changed it to Tatsuo meaning 'dragon boy.' Small in stature by American standards, Shimabuku was only 5' 2" and weighed about 125 pounds. He was a farmer's son and was described as being very practical and intuitive in his dealings in life and with others. Shimabuku was known by many who studied with him as someone who never passed on an opportunity to further his knowledge of the martial arts. He was a karate-ka who respected tradition, but never allowed himself to be bound by it. Shimabuku was known for being a very creative and innovative martial artist.

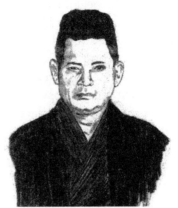

Tatsuo Shimabuku

At the age of six, Shimabuku went to his uncle, Gajoko Chioyu, for lessons in Shuri-te. Initially, Chiyou refused Shimabuku's request and put the young boy to performing tasks such as sweeping, cleaning, and gardening around the dojo. For two years Shimabuku walked six miles to his uncle's dojo only to be refused lessons and then put to work. Finally, when Shimabuku was eight, Chiyou accepted young Shimabuku as a student, and he began his study of the martial arts.

It is believed that Shimabuku studied with Chiyou for four to six years. Chiyou later introduced him to Chotoku Kyan. Kyan instructed Shimabuku in many of the traditional Shurite forms like Wansu, Kusanku, and Chinto. Kyan also gave Shimabuku his first Kobudo lessons. Shimabuku studied with Kyan for somewhere between 15 and 20 years. It was at the young age of 22 when Shimabuku gained fame among Okinawan martial artists for his execution of Chinto kata. This took place before Okinawa's leading martial artists of the day at a festival in Shuri. Shimabuku's fame-winning demonstration lasted less than one minute, yet made him a legend among Okinawan martial artists.

After studying with Chotoku Kyan for many years, Shimabuku began to study Naha-te with Chojun Miyagi where he learned the Seiuchin and Sanchin katas. The exact dates Shimabuku studied under Miyagi are unknown, but he reportedly became one of Miyagi's leading students. Shimabuku's time with Miyagi ended when Miyagi went to China to further his own knowledge of the martial arts. After Miyagi left for China, Shimabuku began studying Shuri-te again with Choki Motobu, a man noted for his fighting abilities. It can be said that Motobu brought forth in Shimabuku some of the more combative overtones present in Isshin-ryu today. It was also somewhere dur-

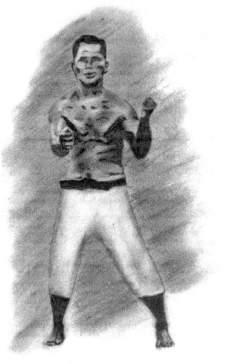

Tatsuo Shimabuku performing Kata.

ing this period when Shimabuku began his study of Kobudo under Taira Shinken. Shimabuku would trade karate lessons with Shinken in return for Kobudo instruction. Their friendship allegedly lasted until Shinken's death in 1970.

By 1940, Shimabuku had begun teaching his own form of karate, and although the system had no official name, it was a blend of both Goju-ryu and Shorin-ryu. At this point in Shimabuku's life, his reputation as a martial artist had grown to where he was known throughout the Ryukyu Islands. By day Shimabuku farmed and ran a small business, and during the evenings he practiced and taught his karate. Then, as fate would have it, an event happened that would alter the slow pace of Ryukyuan society, change Shimabuku's life forever (along with course of his karate,) and lay waste to most of Okinawa. On December 7, 1941 Japanese forces bombed Pearl Harbor, and the following day America declared war on Japan. The Second World War had begun.

On April 1, 1945, 60,000 American soldiers, sailors, and Marines stormed Okinawa, landing on the southwestern portion of the island north of Shuri, between the villages of Chatan and Hagahama. This was the beginning of the largest battle of the Pacific war. It lasted for 83 days, and over 11,000 American military personnel lost their lives. 110,000 Japanese soldiers died, and close to 150,000 Okinawans perished due to starvation or sickness. Although the battle consumed all of Okinawa, the majority of fighting was concentrated in the southern portion of the island around the cities of Shuri and Naha, both of which were completely destroyed during the battle. Many of Okinawa's best karate-ka perished during the war.

The Okinawan population as a whole was against the war. Due to their unpleasant history with the Japanese, the Okinawans were not fully behind them. Nonetheless, many Okinawans were forced into military duty to fight the invading Americans. One day before the invasion, 14 year-old middle school children attending graduation in Shuri were given their junior high diplomas and draft notices at the same ceremony. Some Okinawans chose not to fight, and thus placed their lives in danger by avoiding the Japanese army. Tatsuo Shimabuku was one of these people.

Shimabuku did not support the war, and rather than compromise his moral beliefs and values, he fled. Shimabuku's reputation as a karate-ka haunted him during these years, making him a valuable prize to be had by the Japanese. No matter how hard they tried to catch him however, Shimabuku always seemed to outsmart the army. The war years were hard on all Okinawans, and Shimabuku was no exception. His own father was killed during bombing raids by American planes, and his life on the run took its toll. To end his life as a fugitive, Shimabuku struck a deal with commanding Japanese officers—in exchange for his teaching them karate, Shimabuku was allowed to keep his freedom and remain a civilian.

On June 22, 1945 the battle for Okinawa ended. Although the commanding officer of Japanese forces on the island committed ritual suicide (*hari-kiri*), operations continued for days. Most of the Okinawan population was put in refugee camps set up by the American forces. Life after the war for Okinawans was a constant struggle for survival, as disease and starvation were commonplace. Some Okinawans were employed by the American Army to dig ditches and clear rubble. A great many more turned to the fields and farming. Shimabuku was broke and homeless. The war had taken everything from him, so he returned to farming and attempted to rebuild his life as best as he could. He also returned to practicing his karate. He taught for free because very few Okinawans at that time had money. For seven years after the war, Shimabuku taught on an informal basis, and his reputation as a karate master again began to grow.

By the early 1950's, Shimabuku again began teaching publicly in the village of Chun, but this time things were different. There were thousands of American troops stationed on Okinawa, and it was during this period when Shimabuku gained notoriety among the Americans at the karate demonstration described earlier. During the early fifties, several things happened to bring greater recognition to Shimabuku and his karate. One was his formalization of Isshin-ryu and his adopting the Mizugami or 'water goddess' as the symbol of his karate. Shimabuku's dojo was more of an open field than an actual school. Most training was conducted in his yard, surrounded by the field and paddies he farmed. It was in this very secluded area that American service men began to seek out Shimabuku for instruction.

The popularity of karate slowly began to grow among American service men stationed on Okinawa. Their exposure to the fighting arts came in many forms. One of the most common methods was when drunken, boisterous GI's received on-the-spot instruction from the fast hands and feet of

Okinawan martial artists. During the early years of the occupation, Shimabuku, as with many other Okinawans, was fascinated by the Americans' size. It can be safely assumed that more than one Okinawan karate-ka allowed himself to be drawn into a fight in order to test his technique on such a strapping specimen.

The highly effective methods of combat practiced by the Okinawans soon gained the attention of commanding officers in the American forces. It wasn't long before Okinawan masters were hired by the American military to teach the GI's stationed there. Tatsuo Shimabuku was one of the people employed by the military. Shimabuku soon moved to Agena where he opened up another dojo. He was paid $300 a month (a substantial sum of money back then) by the military to teach local service men.

Many people have discussed the fact that there was a great deal of animosity towards Shimabuku by other Okinawan karate-ka. This may be true, but the tradition of founding one's own system of karate in the Okinawan fighting arts dates back long before Shimabuku's time. Another reason some may have held some animosity toward him was because, up until now, there had been very few full time, "professional" karate instructors in Okinawan history. During the time Okinawa was recovering from the war, money was short, and Shimabuku's position as karate instructor for the military was solidified even more by the fact that he was one of the first hired. It probably didn't hurt matters much that some of his students like Steve Armstrong held key positions at local bases. These individuals were able to direct more business towards Shimabuku. They told new personnel about him, and encouraged them to go to Shimabuku because the lessons were already paid for. On a business level, this made competition against Shimabuku almost nonexistent. This was, no doubt, one of the reasons that competitors were a bit hostile. Although there were other dojos instructing American service men, few were paid by the military to do so.

Many of the original Marines who studied with Shimabuku described his method of teaching as relaxed, yet one which pushed the students to their limits. His method of teaching had no formal beginning or end. Shimabuku would sit cross-legged observing the class, sometimes reading a newspaper and smoking a cigarette. He gave instruction where it was needed. Most of the instruction for lower-ranking belts was given by senior students. Shimabuku's own workout usually began in the early morning with practice of charts one and two, spending up to three hours on them. After this, he would strike the makiwara board, and eventually begin spending a considerable amount of time practicing foot techniques. Shimabuku thought of foot techniques as the element of surprise in combat. Anyone who has seen the film of Shimabuku performing kata will note that his kicking techniques are extremely fast and agile. Shimabuku strived for uniform movement while training and would practice both Kobudo and empty-handed kata during workouts. He was considered an expert with all weapons of the Kobudo system, but was especially noted for his Bo-jutsu technique.

Its been said that the Agena dojo is where Isshin-ryu was finally solidified as a system, but even after relocating to Agena, Shimabuku was constantly experimenting with Isshin-ryu. He was constantly adding or subtracting techniques, and always striving to better his style of karate. By the early 1960's, Shimabuku and Isshin-ryu's fame had spread not only among Marines stationed on Okinawa, but in the United States as well. This was due to the fact that some of the Marines stationed on Okinawa were rotating stateside and subsequently opening their own Isshin-ryu dojos. It was around this time that current problems so prevalent in the Isshin-ryu system were first brought up. Because there were no appointed figureheads or governing organizations over Isshin-ryu in the United States, standards varied from one individual to another. In most cases, before departing Okinawa, Shimabuku told the future Isshin-ryu instructor to teach in the manner which they felt was the most effective. Some people have questioned this line of thinking, but it is important to take into consideration that Shimabuku was obviously not familiar with American culture. Perhaps one can conclude that Shimabuku put faith in these future teachers to present their knowledge in a manner more appropriate for American Isshin-ryu students.

During the early 1960's, Shimabuku made several trips to America hosted by his Marine students. It was during one of his last visits in 1966 that Shimabuku was filmed performing empty-handed and Kobudo Isshin-ryu katas as they were being taught and practiced at the time. As mentioned earlier, this tape would later become the absolute final word on Isshin-ryu for many practitioners. Others, however, would interpret Shimabuku's performance more liberally. It was also during this last visit when Shimabuku appointed Steve Armstrong, Harold Long, and Don Nagle to govern Isshin-ryu in the United States. Appointing three leaders has been questioned by many over the years, and it has caused much confusion and animosity within the Isshin-ryu ranks. Many have faulted Shimabuku for the resulting mess. When we look at Isshin-ryu as it stands today, with its various political organizations, perhaps we should blame ourselves instead of Tatsuo Shimabuku. In many cases we have allowed Isshin-ryu to become fragmented due to our own egos and personal quests for fame and power and not, as many claim, due to the appointment of three American figure heads.

Tatsuo Shimabuku died on May 30th, 1975 at the age of 67. He never left a text on how Isshin-ryu should be taught, or appointed one distinctive figurehead to preside over the whole system. Although some may disagree, one can argue that Shimabuku did in fact leave an outline (albeit a broad one) for the practice of Isshin-ryu karate. This is evident by some of the contrasts in technique of the earlier Isshin-ryu practitioners, and those who studied shortly with him before his death. Although there are differences in technique within the kata, *the basic principles remain relatively unchanged.* Had there been no standardization at all, the techniques would have certainly changed drastically over the years.

Several theories exist about why Shimabuku left his system "up in the air." Perhaps it was left this way so practitioners would be forced to look within themselves to further its development. The Isshin-ryu pioneers knew Shimabuku was not afraid to experiment in developing his karate. This practice today is more or less taboo in dojos. In our own attempts to standardize a system, we may be stifling creativity and end up producing clones rather than true martial artists. Others say that Shimabuku realized Isshin-ryu would splinter into many groups, as had been the case with other systems before it, so he simply did not see the point in organizing a governing body. Still another, less talked-about theory, is that Shimabuku planned on leaving a master text to be followed, but died before he could do so.

Consider how the evolution of Isshin-ryu would have been effected if Shimabuku left a set format. It would have made us lazy, turned us away from our own creativity, and left to rely on a set of rules which would be interpreted to the letter when a question arose. Instead, Isshin-ryu practitioners have to rely upon themselves for answers. This certainly causes its share of problems, but in the long run it will only help Isshin-ryu to evolve into an effective, more personal art for its practitioners than Shimabuku could have ever imagined.

CHAPTER 8

Isshin-Ryu's Code of Ethics

Today's Isshin-ryu karate-ka can only guess what Tatsuo
Shimabuku's reasons were for organizing the system the way
he did. There's an old saying that says the body must be able
to change direction at any time. With this in mind, Isshin-ryu
practitioners should perhaps accept the organization of Isshin-
ryu as it is. All we can really do is to be flexible, respect our
fellow Isshin-ryu practitioner's views, and continue onward in
our practice and development. The only written guide left by
Shimabuku is the eight-point Isshin-ryu code. This code is a
philosophical outlook not only on the fighting strategies of
Isshin-ryu, but the spiritual aspects of the system as well. The
code is as follows:

1. A person's heart is the same as heaven and earth.
2. The blood circulating is similar to the sun and moon.
3. A manner of drinking and spitting is neither hard or
   soft.
4. A person's unbalance is the same as weight.
5. The body should be able to change direction at anytime.
6. The time to strike is when the opportunity presents
   itself.
7. The eye must see all sides.
8. The ear must listen in all directions.

There are many interpretations of the Isshin-ryu code with
each one varying among individuals. Some are of a more literal sense, while others tend to be more of a philosophical
nature. The Isshin-ryu code is much like Musashi's classic *Book
of Five Rings*. Miyamoto Musashi was Japan's greatest swords-
man, and his classical text on strategy and battle has many
different interpretations and translations. Many of the inter-

pretations within Shimabuku's eight-point code will change as a practitioner matures in karate and in life. Listed are a few of the common interpretations of each of the eight points in the Isshin-ryu code.

1. **A person's heart is the same as heaven and earth.**
   - There are certain limitations placed upon man while in his physical state, but there are no such limitations to his spiritual development. There are qualities of heaven and earth within each person and because of this, humans are the strongest and weakest creatures in the universe.
   - The Isshin-ryu practitioner should strive to be in harmony with all things great and small.
   - The life force or energy within each human is the same as all other forms of life. The energy of nature and man are one in the same.

2. **The blood circulating is similar to the moon and sun.**
   - Energy in motion remains in motion, and stillness brings forth dullness in body and spirit.
   - Under the right circumstances, human nature is as reliable as the orbits of the sun and moon. Take notice of another's nature and trust it within yourself.
   - During the course of one's life, a person should always be flexible and mobile. When an obstacle is encountered they will yield and pass by, never clash head-on and break.

3. **The manner of drinking and spitting is either hard or soft.**
   - In terms of combative technique, there is no hard or soft. There is no right way or wrong way—only what works for the practitioner.
   - In the course of one's life, a person's character will be both soft and passive, or hard and unyielding. It will change from time to time. Neither way is right or wrong, both are merely different paths with the same end result

4. **A person's unbalance is the same as a weight.**
   - Balance, be it physical or mental, is crucial in defeating an opponent and overcoming life's obstacles. A

person without balance trying to overcome an obstacle will only find the task twice as difficult.

- There must be harmony between mind and body. The two elements must be of equal proportion, combined together into a whole unit, with one unified train of thought uncluttered by excess mental projections.

5. **The body should be able to change direction at any time.**

- You should be able to respond to any threat, attack, or event in a natural manner without any anticipation or hesitation.

- From a combative aspect, the body should be able to utilize any and all forms of movement while fighting an opponent.

- The practitioner should be able to adapt to any situation they find themselves in and, at the same time, have the ability to overcome any obstacle.

6. **The time to strike is when opportunity presents itself.**

- Timing is crucial to almost any endeavor in life. The time to act, be it in a crisis or everyday routine, is at the proper moment. Do not act too quickly or too slowly, but at the proper time so your actions will have the most desired results.

- From a combative aspect, strike your opponent at their weakest moment or at weakest point.

7. **The eye must see all sides.**

- To clearly understand a subject, a person must learn to view matters from all angles. He must look at and respect others' views.

- From a combative aspect, this can be translated as focusing on your opponent's outline, and not one singular portion of their body. Doing this allows you to see every movement executed.

- You must not only be able to notice and understand other people's emotions, but your own as well.

8. **The ear must listen in all directions.**

- A person has to understand not only his analytical tendencies to rationalize and theorize, but also his intuition.

- Many times you will hear your opponent before seeing him. This is especially true with attacks from behind. Where your eyes cannot see, you must cover that area with your hearing.

Whether Shimabuku's eight-point code was influenced by an Asian philosophy or manuscript on strategy such as Sun Tzu's *Art of War*, has yet to be determined. This is a possibility, although one must remember that Buddhism did not heavily influence Okinawan karate. After reading this code however, it is very easy to see how many people could make such an assumption. Many of the ideals expressed by Shimabuku can also be found in various religions and philosophies. The Isshin-ryu code simply appears to have been Shimabuku's own personal guidelines for living. The eight points set forth for the Isshin-ryu system evolved as a result of his own personal experiences in karate, life, and that place within everyone's soul where the two overlap. It should be kept in mind the Isshin-ryu code is not a text of mystical enlightenment containing supernatural overtones or mystical powers. It should not be made into something it is not. The code is simply a guide for strategy and everyday life—one to be interpreted by the practitioner's own intuition and logic. Shimabuku is also credited for having written another set of guidelines for karate. This was the called the "dojo oath" and it is a code of conduct the practitioner should abide by while in the dojo. Like the Isshin-ryu eight-point code, the dojo oath can also be used as a guideline for conducting oneself in everyday life. The oath itself is a bit more literal in its translation and reads as follows:

1. We will train our hearts and bodies for a firm, unshaking spirit.
2. We will pursue the true meaning of the martial way.
3. With true vigor, will seek to cultivate a spirit of self-denial.
4. We will observe the rules of courtesy, respect our superiors, and refrain from violence.
5. We will pay homage to our creator and never forget the true virtue of humility.
6. We will look upwards to wisdom and strength and not seek other desires.

7. All our lives, through the discipline of karate, we will seek to fulfill the true meaning of the Way.

Still a third creed often used in the arts is something called, "the karate creed." Tatsuo Shimabuku did not write this, and it is a philosophy adopted by many systems of both Japanese and Okinawan karate. It is used in many Isshin-ryu dojos along with Shimabuku's dojo oath, and the eight-point code. One of the karate creeds' purposes is to instill a higher sense of morality within the karate-ka. The karate creed also parallels the fourth and sixth points of the Isshin-ryu code. For example, the sixth point states that the time to strike is when the opportunity presents itself. The creed echoes this and provides more guidance along that line:

The Karate Creed. I come to you with only karate— Empty Hands. I have no weapons, but should I be forced to defend myself, my principles, or my honor—should it be a matter of life or death, right or wrong, then here are my weapons—Karate—my Empty Hands.

On some occasions karate-ka will strike an opponent out of anger. This is done not because they have been threatened or endangered, but because they've simply became angry. This goes against the karate creed as well as the fourth point of the Isshin-ryu code, which states a person's unbalance is the same as a weight. From a mental standpoint, if you're angry, you will be unable to engage an opponent as effectively as you would in a calm, rational state of mind. Anger causes a person to loose control and when this happens, much of the karate-ka's training and technique is thrown to the wind. There are many spiritual and physical avenues of study inherent in the Isshin-ryu system. Philosophical aspects are important to not only Isshin-ryu but to all systems. They add that extra depth to our training and make us ask ourselves, "what if?" Philosophy helps us look at our training from a more abstract view, and provides the depth that simple physical training cannot. The fourth point of the Isshin-ryu code focuses on a person's unbalance. There must be a balance between philosophy and technique. Many practitioners will delve into the philosophical aspects of the martial arts so deeply that they lose sight of the physical aspects of the system they are studying. In doing so, many practitioners will consider the study of technique secondary to their philosophical quest for something which may or may not exist...

This philosophical quest is happening to many martial systems these days, especially those like Aikido and Tai Chi. Isshin-ryu has not avoided this trend completely, as we have our own share of philosophers. Philosophical aspects and techniques go hand-in-hand, and provide an excellent system of checks and balances. The physical techniques of the martial arts are quite dangerous and certainly not something to be taken lightly. The grandmasters of the arts knew this and, along with teaching physical technique, taught and upheld a high standard of ethics that helps karate-ka from turning their techniques upon helpless individuals. Isshin-ryu is a martial art as well as a science of self- defense, and self-development. It is not a college course on enlightenment, as some practitioners would like to have us believe.

CHAPTER 9

The Principles of
Isshin-Ryu Karate

Like most other martial arts, Isshin-ryu has its own distinctive principles and features. The most notable may be its
vertical punch with the thumb positioned on top of the fist.
This particular technique is what most people associate with
Isshin-ryu. There are other features of the system as well.
Depending upon the dojo or organization a practitioner
belongs to, there can be anywhere from 10 to 15 other principles used to define Isshin-ryu. It is important to note, however, that the interpretation of these principles may differ
between dojos. As we learned earlier, no one system of
Okinawan karate is entirely hard or soft. The various aspects
of a system and how they are taught will vary from teacher to
teacher. Listed below are some of Isshin-ryu's principles.

1. All techniques are based on rapid and natural movement.
2. Strikes are with maximum power and minimum effort.
3. Elimination of artistically appealing techniques and
   movements.
4. A balance of opposites. The body is soft until contact
   is made with the opponent. At that moment, the body
   becomes hard and all energy is focused into one point.
5. Vertical punch with the thumb on top.
6. Offensive and defensive techniques are executed with
   naturally hardened or padded portions of the body.
7. Sanchin should be practiced often, as it aids in the
   development of meditation, breath control, and proper body tension.
8. All movement centers on a point located 1.25 inches
   (3 cm.) below the navel. This is the center of the body
   and is referred to in Chinese as the tantien.

9. The trigger for all movement is proper breathing.

10. Use of low kicks below solar plexus level.

11. Snapping punches and kicks.

12. Hand and foot techniques are 50/50. In some dojos, the ratio is closer to 70/30.

13. All techniques can be used in a variety of situations.

14. Equal balance and mobility should be maintained in all directions.

15. Offense and defense are one.

Shimabuku was exposed to a great deal of knowledge over the course of his life. He witnessed first-hand much of the evolution of Okinawan karate. There is an old saying regarding karate that there is no new knowledge, only knowledge that is forgotten and later rediscovered. Shimabuku learned a tremendous amount from his instructors, but he later took that knowledge, expanded it, and made it his own. Embedded within Isshin-ryu's features are Okinawan Te, Chinese influences, and the Shuri and Naha-te fighting methods. Most systems of Okinawan arts are of a combative nature and designed to eliminate an opponent as quickly and effectively as possible, not score points or plot strategies for three-minute rounds. Let us examine some of Isshin-ryu's basic features and principles in greater detail.

All techniques are based on rapid and natural movement. The techniques, stances, and footwork of Isshin-ryu are all designed to allow the karate-ka's body to move in a fluid manner, without the body's parts working against one another during the course of movement, or in a way which would cause injury to the practitioner.

Strikes are with maximum power and minimum effort. The goal of each technique is to strike with maximum power using minimum effort. The Chinese have a saying, "Big movements are not as polished as small movements, small movements are not as polished as stillness." The development of proper body mechanics is a must for the martial artist. It is imperative to be able to capitalize off the slightest or smallest movement. Aside from helping to develop proper body mechanics, Isshin-ryu is a system of small, economical movements. There are no large, lunging-type techniques that may be found in other systems such as Shotokan. Isshin-ryu has no intricate hand movements that are found in some Chinese systems. Instead all techniques within Isshin-ryu are based on economy of motion.

Elimination of artistically appealing techniques and movements. It has been said that all techniques within Isshin-ryu can be utilized as they are shown in the kata and that little or no modification is needed by the practitioner. Other forms of karate and Chinese boxing may have movements in their kata that are *symbolic* of true combat techniques, but may require the stylist to dig deeper to find the true application. Still other kata may be artistically appealing and help develop physical dexterity as opposed to drilling combat technique. Artistic techniques are not found in Isshin-ryu. All techniques are to be performed as they are practiced. Isshin-ryu's strong points are its simplicity, subtleness, and effectiveness.

A balance of opposites. The practitioner's body should be relaxed to facilitate fluid, faster movements, better concentration, and natural breathing. The moment the practitioner strikes an opponent, there is an exhalation of air and the practitioner's body tenses; the result of which is a whip-like action. Speed and momentum are turned into power and multiplied as the strike reaches maximum velocity by the tensing of the body. This tensing, or "state of Sanchin" lasts only for a split-second and allows the practitioners body to return to a relaxed state once again. Many other systems of the martial arts utilize this method of generating power as well. Bruce Lee was a master of this technique and would constantly amaze people by knocking over four or five large men with his "one-inch" and "three-inch" punches.

The use of the vertical punch with the thumb on top. This type of strike can be traced back to the early days of Okinawan Te. The vertical fist is said to be one of the few punching methods that would actually penetrate the armor of the samurai. Many types of modern day karate utilize a twisting-type punch. This technique was added when karate was introduced into the Okinawan public schools in the earlier part of the century. The twisting was thought to be safer for students to practice as it would reduce the possibility of injury.

Isshin-ryu strikes are made with a vertical punch, palm inward, the thumb on top of the fist. This position greatly adds to the power generated in the punching arm and wrist has much less of a tendency to buckle. Isshin-ryu is not the only system of martial arts to employ such a method of punching. Burmese Bando, along with many Chinese systems of fighting, are also noted for having vertical punches within their arsenals.

Offensive and defensive techniques are executed with naturally hardened or padded portions of the body. No bone-meet-bone type blocks are executed in Isshin-ryu. Defensive techniques are executed using the muscular portions of the arm and all strikes are performed using the naturally hardened areas of the body such as the first two knuckles of the hand or ball of the foot. Striking with these areas greatly reduces the risk of the practitioner injuring himself when blocking or striking. Blocking with the muscular portions of the arm also greatly enhances the softer, circular aspects of many Isshin-ryu blocking techniques.

Sanchin should be practiced often as it aids in the development of meditation, breath control, and proper body tension. Sanchin has been called the backbone of Isshin-ryu karate. Sanchin helps develop all elements of Isshin-ryu and combines them into one functioning unit. Along with its other benefits, Sanchin develops dynamic tension (an important part of body mechanics in Isshin-ryu) as well as helps cultivate the karate-ka's chi. Sanchin is practiced in the Uechi and Goju systems of karate as well.

All movement centers on a point located 1.25 inches (3 cm.) below the navel. Over a period of time and continuous practice, the karate-ka's center of gravity should begin to settle lower, eventually sinking into this abdominal region where many believe the reservoir of a person's chi (internal energy) is located. The Japanese consider this area the center of a man's being—the focal point of his own universe. When a karate-ka's center does finally settle into this region, all movement and action will be that much more powerful and stable.

The trigger for all movement is proper breathing. The Chinese say, "The air is the lord of strength." This is especially true when referring to the martial arts. The effectiveness of both offensive and defensive techniques revolve around a practitioner's breathing. Upon inhaling, the body should relax and the center of gravity should drop. It is at this point when most defensive techniques are performed. When the martial artist exhales, forcing all air from the lungs, it aids in developing proper tension and power. This is the moment when most offensive techniques are performed.

In later stages of development, the practitioner learns how to reverse these roles. Without proper breathing practice however, one physical techniques will not be effective as they could be. This is one of the reasons why Sanchin practice is stressed so much within the Isshin-ryu system. Rhythmic forms of breathing are common in many martial arts. They aid in developing proper focus and help one attain a calm, 'Zen' state of mind. Proper breathing also aids in helping to achieve and maintain good stamina, a must for any martial artist.

Use of low kicks below solar plexus level. Unlike many systems of karate that utilize flying kicks and foot techniques to the head, Isshin-ryu does not. One of the most basic combative principles is to strike a target with the weapon closest to it. Kicking techniques in Isshin-ryu are often aimed at targets below the opponents waist, simply because the legs are closer to this area than the hands are. Hand techniques are concentrated on areas above the opponent's waist.

Mobility is essential in combat and anytime you kick, your body is (if only for a split second) stationary. Since kicks to head level leave you stationary longer, they stand a greater chance of being intercepted or trapped by an opponent—certainly not ideal in a combat situation.

Snapping punches and kicks. This ties in with the third principle that refers to the body remaining soft until contact with the target. There are very few thrusting foot or hand techniques in Isshin-ryu. Most techniques are based on the "snap" principle. This takes less muscular force to execute and relies more upon body mechanics and proper form to achieve a more explosive type of power.

Hand and foot techniques are 50/50. In some dojos, the ratio is closer to 70/30. Since the Isshin-ryu practitioner does a lot of his fighting close-up, foot techniques are used in a supportive role. Fighting at close range enables the karate-ka to finish off the aggressor with hand techniques. The heavy reliance on hands could also be due to the earlier influence of Te and Chinese methods of fighting on Isshin-ryu.

All techniques can be used in a variety of situations. Many of the blocks within Isshin-ryu can be used as strikes to the opponent's limbs and body. By utilizing multi-purpose strikes and blocks, the effectiveness of techniques within the Isshin-ryu system is doubled. Further, the distinction between what is offensive and defensive diminishes.

Equal balance and mobility should be maintained in all directions. Equal balance and mobility should be maintained in all directions. This principle is also related to the fifth principle of the Isshin-ryu code, which states that the body should be able to change direction at any time. In order to be an effective combatant, the practitioner must maintain balance and mobility. Without these two elements you cannot and will not be able to engage an opponent. If you are immobile and constantly off balance, your opponent will undoubtedly be able to do some damage.

Offense and defense are one. This is a statement many will disagree with and others will wholeheartedly support. It is related to the 13th principle that discusses the importance of multi-purpose techniques. In many cases, the distinguishing factor between offense and defense is non-existent. For instance, if your opponent punches and you strike his punching arm before it hits you, was your strike defensive or offensive?

Much of the confusion surrounding what constitutes offense or defense has to do with timing. In the beginning of a karate-ka's studies, he has very little concept of what timing is, and thinks in terms of 'attack' and 'defend.' Beginners will punch then cover, but never perform the two actions simultaneously. As the student develops however, he gains a sense of timing that allows him to perform techniques not merely in an offensive/defensive mode, but as counters as well. Eventually, the practitioner will mature to the point when they come to think of offense and defense as one in the same.

Each system of karate has its own particular features and stylistic differences. Shotokan, for example, is known to be a linear, strong, straightforward method of karate whereas Aikido is known for its circular movements and its joint locking techniques. In some cases, the similarities between arts may overlap. This is particularly true with Isshin-ryu and other Okinawan fighting arts. The evolution of a particular art, and the characteristics that come to be associated with it, is due to the progression of the martial arts as a whole, the small size of Okinawa, and the constant interplay between various styles, teachers, and students when the arts were being developed. Awareness of how the characteristics of our own chosen art came about can only help us further our own progress, both mentally and physically, as martial artists.

CHAPTER 10

Mizugami—The Symbol of Isshin-Ryu Karate

The Mizugami is the patch worn on the left breast of the Isshin-ryu practitioner's gi. It is the symbol of Isshin-ryu karate and some consider it the missing link in the final formation of Isshin-ryu. There are two versions of the Mizugami patch. One is oval with an orange border while the other is formed more like a vertical fist. There is a lot of symbolism surrounding the Mizugami. Some say the patch represents Okinawan folklore and history. Others look at the emblem and see the essence of Isshin-ryu and the Okinawan martial arts philosophies.

The woman on the patch is a Shinto water goddess known as Mizugami. The idea for the patch originated in a dream that Shimabuku had just prior to his formalization of Isshin-ryu as a system. In his dream, a man confronted him and, although Shimabuku felt no threat or danger from the stranger, he waved him on with an open hand to show peaceful intentions, but kept his other fist closed. This represented his willingness to fight if need be. This is the same position as the Mizugami's hands in the patch.

Eventually, the man departed, but before doing so he surrounded Shimabuku with a wall of flames, and it is from this point on that two conflicting stories are told. One story says that Shimabuku himself put out the flames, the another says that the Water Goddess extinguished the flames herself. In either case it is the Mizugami which was eventually chosen by Shimabuku to be symbolic of Isshin-ryu karate. In 1960 Shimabuku talked about his dream to James Advincula, a young Marine studying Isshin-ryu at the time. It was Advincula who is credited with designing the original Mizugami.

The Oval-like Shape of the Patch

A. This represents the Isshin-ryu vertical fist.
B. The circular shape may also point to the fact that Isshin-ryu is a complete system that encompasses all aspects of the martial arts.
C. There is no beginning or end, only a continuous journey in one's perfection.

Mizugami

A. The water goddess symbolizes the calm a martial artist should have in the face of danger. Her left hand is open signifying peace, and her right is closed showing her determination to fight if necessary.
B. The turbulent water around her represents the troubles in life everyone will encounter. It can also signify the focused power of karate-ka.

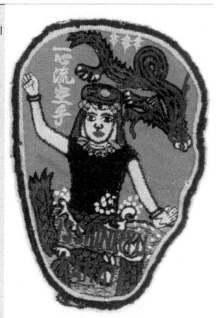

Mizugami Patch

Three Stars

A. The three stars may represent Shorin-ryu, Goju-ryu, and Kobudo; the three systems that make up Isshin-ryu.
B. Shorin-ryu, Goju-ryu are the 'mother' and 'father' systems and child born from them is Isshin-ryu.
C. Chotoku Kyan, Chojun Miyagi, and Choki Motobu three of Shimabuku's instructors.

The patch itself is oval in shape. One version is bordered by orange, the other by yellow. It is the yellow-bordered patch that looks a bit like a vertical fist. The Mizugami sits in the middle of a gray sky, her right hand clenched in a fist, the left is open. The lower half of her body is submerged in a rough choppy sea, and above her is a dragon. At the top of the patch, above the dragon, are three stars.

Like many other things in Isshin-ryu, there are various interpretations of the symbols on the patch. The following is a list of some of the more common interpretations of the Mizugami:

These are just a few interpretations of the Mizugami. It must be kept in mind that many are individual interpretations of the Mizugami. To one person, a certain translation may

D. There are three aspects of Isshin-ryu—the hard, the soft, and the middle element that is a combination of the two.
E. The three stars can also represent the evening, a time during early Okinawan history when most Okinawans trained in order to avoid detection by the Japanese.

Orange Border
A. Signifies the wall of flame that encircled Shimabuku in his dream
B. Represents a higher state of enlightenment, self-realization, or spiritual power that can be attained through the practice of karate.

Dragon
A. Dragons have always been symbols of good luck in Okinawan culture. The dragon may show that those who study Isshin-ryu will prosper from the benefits of studying karate.
B. The Dragon can also represent Shimabuku, the 'Dragon Boy' founder of Isshin-ryu.
C. The inner fury or fighting spirit of a karate-ka.

Gray Sky
A. The inner calm of the martial artist.
B. A void or emptiness. Through the practice of Isshin-ryu you should try to empty yourself of all egotistical and self-defeating tendencies and strive to have serenity within.
C. The emptiness of all emotion. This state should be reflected by the karate-ka to his opponent while engaged in conflict. The karate-ka's face should be empty yet polished as a mirror reflecting the opponent's greatest fears back to them.

have little or no significance, but to another it may bear much knowledge and foresight. The interpretations of the Mizugami, like the principles of Isshin-ryu, are much like studying a martial art. They become endeavors that in time evolve into personal translations best suited to the practitioners needs.

As it stands now, there is already a 'loose' sense of uniformity to the Mizugami's interpretations, the Isshin-ryu code, and Isshin-ryu karate itself. This flexible framework was brought forth by Isshin-ryu's history, its physical characteristics, and Tatsuo Shimabuku's teachings. This flexibility makes for much bickering within the Isshin-ryu ranks. However, to take away this element of personal growth and experimentation would also take away much of the creativity in Isshin-ryu. It is this creativity which allows the system to grow and add new knowledge and ideals. It does not allow the system to stagnate like so many others that have extremely stringent guidelines.

As mentioned above, one implication of the Mizugami's oval shape is that Isshin-ryu is a whole system. If this is true, then that means each Isshin-ryu karate-ka has room for his own growth within the system. Each has room to experiment and find what best suits him, both physically and philosophically, within Isshin-ryu.

Like the Mizugami's interpretations, Isshin-ryu encompasses far more than we would like to admit at times. Instead of looking for absolutes in our training and constantly asking ourselves what Isshin-ryu is, maybe we would better serve ourselves (and the system as a whole) if we look more deeply and ask ourselves what Isshin-ryu is not.

CHAPTER 11

Empty-Handed Kata
of Isshin-Ryu

When translated into English, the word *kata* literally means 'form.' Almost all martial arts have some concept of prearranged fighting forms in their teachings. Throughout the years, kata has been one of the traditional methods of teaching and practicing many martial arts. The practice of kata is very beneficial in that it allows the karate-ka to practice a certain sequence of techniques or movements in a uniform fashion until perfection has been achieved. Kata practice also helps develop coordination, body mechanics, the lowering of one's center, and concentration. Kata also allows the practitioner to execute techniques with full power. If these same techniques were practiced with someone and a mistake was made, serious injury would be the inevitable result. The training methods of Okinawan Kobudo and karate prior to WWII relied heavily upon kata and prearranged sparring forms. After the war, free sparring became a widely accepted means of practice. To reduce the risk of endangering contestants, padded equipment was introduced and some techniques were modified. This took away from the students' effectiveness, but also reduced the risk of injury.

The role kata plays in the martial arts is a hotly debated subject. It is made more complicated by the growing popularity of sport karate where the practice of kata is done more for competition than for combative or martial training. It is not uncommon to see many traditional forms being completely discarded and replaced by very acrobatic forms designed to win tournaments. This practice has begun to find its way into Isshin-ryu as well. It depends upon the dojo naturally, but Isshin-ryu kata have been performed in such acrobatic and flamboyant ways that would put Jackie Chan in awe. However, there are still many dojos where the Isshin-ryu kata are practiced with a more down to earth approach. As guidelines for their practice, these practitioners use the code of Isshin-ryu, the film of Tatsuo Shimabuku, or numerous manuscripts that have been published over the years by Isshin-ryu karate-ka.

Isshin-ryu contains empty-handed kata from both Shuri-te and Naha-te systems, as well as Kobudo kata. There are many similarities between the empty-handed kata of Isshin-ryu and the original form. For example, while Seiuchin is performed almost exactly like the original Goju version, other kata like Wansu or Chinto bare only a very slight resemblance to the original form. If one compares the original Shorin-ryu and Goju katas to their equivalents in Shimabuku's system, the first thing one notices is the economy of movement in Isshin-ryu kata. Some Isshin-ryu versions are shorter, more compact, and perhaps a bit simpler to execute. These differences are all due to Shimabuku's teachings and philosophies that stress, among other things, maximum effectiveness from minimum movement.

There are eight empty-handed katas in the Isshin-ryu system. Five can trace their roots to the Shorin school of Okinawan karate. Two are of Goju origins and the eighth, Sunsu, which translated means 'strong one' or 'dragon boy,' refers to Shimabuku himself. He developed this form which is not found in any other system. The breakdown is as follows:

Shorin-ryu kata
- Seisan
- Naihanchi
- Wansu
- Chinto
- Kusanku

Goju-ryu kata
- Seiuchin
- Sanchin

Isshin-ryu kata
- Sunsu

What follows is a brief summary of the Isshin-ryu empty-handed kata along with some of the more notable traits and characteristics of each form.

Seisan. Seisan and Sanchin are two of the oldest forms in Okinawan karate today. It is not uncommon for these kata to be practiced in the Shuri-te, Tomari-te, and Naha-te schools of karate. These two forms are not only found in Okinawan systems of karate, but in Japanese karate as well. Seisan is commonly practiced in the Shito-ryu, Wado-ryu, and Shotokan styles.

Seisan, or Hangetsu as it is known in Shotokan karate, means 'half moon' and refers to the semi-circular stepping used in the kata that helps develop skill in linear fighting. Seisan teaches the practitioner how to move off line and how to shift one's body from side to side. Isshin-ryu's version of Seisan is similar to other styles, but there are some distinct differences.

The Isshin-ryu Seisan has only one side block at the beginning of the kata which is followed immediately by three reverse punches. Other styles will execute a side block prior to each punch. The Isshin-ryu Seisan also uses a double head block at the end of this first punching sequence, whereas most Shuri-te versions execute a double punch.

Footwork is very similar, but again, there are some exceptions. For example, the Isshin-ryu karate-ka perform their hook blocks in unison with the stepping foot, whereas this sequence is done with opposite hand and foot in the Shotokan, Wado-ryu, and Shorin- ryu versions.

Seiuchin. Seiuchin is the first of two Goju-ryu katas incorporated into the Isshin-ryu system. There is very little difference between the Isshin-ryu and Goju styles of Seiuchin. There are various translations of Seiuchin. One is 'marching far quietly,' others are, 'war kata,' and 'lull in the storm.' Seiuchin drew strong influences from the Pa Kua and Hsing-I systems, both of which were studied by Kanryo Higashionna, the father of Naha-te, and Chojun Miyagi, the father of Goju-ryu.

One of the more notable features of Seiuchin is that there are no kicks, and that most of it is performed from a low stance. Many of the more advanced applications within the kata deal with the grappling aspects of combat such as joint locks, throws, and methods of unbalancing. In addition, there are other aspects that teach the practitioner how to drop below an opponent's attack. From a physical standpoint, the practice of this form is known for developing the karate-ka's leg and thigh muscles, the ability to lower one's center of gravity, and stamina.

Seiuchin is also to be found in other systems of karate. Okinawan Goju-ryu, Japanese Goju-ryu, and Shito-ryu also have the kata in their teachings. In some cases there may be a variance in breathing methods between the systems while performing Seiuchin. Some systems may stress more of a Sanchin method of controlled breathing while performing the kata, while others will utilize more of a natural form of breathing in the kata's execution.

Naihanchi. The purpose of Naihanchi kata in Isshin-ryu is sometimes hotly debated. Many practitioners do not see any meaning in it outside of physical development. Practicing Naihanchi helps build, and gain control of, the body's muscular groups from the waist down. There are practitioners who claim the kata's purpose is to teach technique. Naihanchi is noted for its simultaneous blocking and striking combinations. The kata is very unique in that there is no forward motion. Instead the practitioner moves in a side to side fashion, always staying on the same line. Naihanchi is an excellent form, and there is much to be gained from its practice.

Naihanchi comes from the Shuri-te systems, and was much longer in its original form. Due to the kata's complexity, it was broken down into three segments called Naihanchi one, two and three. Some systems like Shotokan teach all three of the Naihanchi forms, while others teach only one out of the series. Of the three katas in the Naihanchi series, Isshin-ryu's version more closely resembles Naihanchi one.

The name Naihanchi means 'iron horse.' The form was originally called Naifanchi, but was changed by Funakoshi to Tekki when he founded his Shotokan system. Despite the differences in the name however, the form remains basically the same. Two of Naihanchi's more notable practitioners were Choki Motobu and Chotoku Kyan. It is thought that these two men taught the form to Shimabuku, and that he later went on to combine the most useful elements of all three versions into the Isshin-ryu version we see today. One small difference between the Isshin-ryu version of Naihanchi and the other Japanese systems is that the hand movements in the Isshin-ryu system appear somewhat softer and more circular in nature. This is more than likely due to the 'soft' element of Goju-ryu's influences on Shimabuku.

Sanchin. Sanchin's lineage and teachings can be traced to some of the earliest recorded periods of history in the martial arts. The principles of Sanchin were introduced to China by Bodhidharma who journeyed from India to unite the various schools of Buddhism that had emerged in China. Bodhidharma planned to establish a Buddhist monastery, but as fate would have it, his original intentions were side-tracked. Instead, he founded the Shaolin Temple, a place were the seeds of many of today's martial arts were sown, and the original concepts of Sanchin were developed.

Kanryo Higashionna is the man given credit for introducing Sanchin to Okinawan karate. Higashionna was taught this kata by Woo Lu Chin, a Chuan Fa master who Higashionna studied with in Fuchou province in China. Higashionna later taught Sanchin to Chojun Miyagi, and Miyagi passed it on to Shimabuku.

The Isshin-ryu version of Sanchin is somewhat shorter than the Goju version. Depending on how it is performed, the Isshin-ryu version contains between 49 to 53 movements. Goju's version contains around 60 to 65 movements. The main difference between the two is that the Goju version contains an "about face" directly to the practitioner's rear at the end of the reverse punch sequence. The sequence then repeats in the opposite direction. The Isshin-ryu Sanchin does not contain these additional movements.

Sanchin is a method of training that focuses more on developing body and mind than on combative technique. Sanchin is usually where the Isshin-ryu practitioner is first taught the principle of dynamic tension. Although the form is most commonly known for helping a practitioner develop dynamic tension, there are other more meditative aspects inherent as well.

Through a combination of dynamic tension, controlled

breathing, and movement, Sanchin is said to bring together body and mind in one functioning unit. There is, however, a debate over the teaching and practice of Sanchin. Many believe it is essential to practice the kata every day with full power in order to achieve maximum results. Others feel that, because the kata is so intense physically, Sanchin should only be practiced with full intensity only once or twice a week at the most. Some believe that daily practice of this kata can place enormous amounts of strain and pressure on the lungs, stomach, and intestines. There is yet another school of thought developing that stresses the practice of Sanchin as purely a breathing kata with no emphasis on dynamic tension. In this form, Sanchin is performed in a slow, rhythmic way in conjunction with the practitioners breathing. There is no tension present in the practitioner's limbs, and the body stays soft and relaxed. Regardless of interpretation, however, most will unanimously agree that that this kata should not, under any circumstances, be taught to young adults who have not yet reached the age of puberty for fear the kata may place too much strain on their bodies.

Sanchin, like so many other aspects of the martial arts, has evolved greatly over time. It will more than likely continue to evolve in the future. How the kata is taught, what its intrinsic value is, and what points are emphasized in training will also change. No matter how it is practiced however, Sanchin is a valuable tool for the practitioner, a tool that develops many essential assets for the karate-ka's total development and evolution.

Wansu. Wansu's lineage in Okinawan karate can be traced back about three hundred years to the days of early Te. It is believed that the principles and techniques contained in Wansu were introduced to Okinawan martial arts by a Chinese military attaché named Wansu. In some forms of Japanese karate (Shotokan, for instance) the kata is also known as Empi or 'flying swallow.' The Japanese name refers to a sequence of techniques where the practitioner responds to an upper-level attack by moving in and around, grasps the attacker's arm pulling him inward, and then counterstriking. The body's motion in this series of movements resembles those of a sparrow in flight. This is much the same as the body movements executed during open-arch-sweep-gouge series in the Isshin-ryu Wansu kata. Shimabuku changed Wansu's original name to its present form before incorporating it into the Isshin-ryu system. Wansu means 'dumping form,' and refers to the hip throw that comes midway through the kata. This movement is probably the signature technique of Wansu.

Another very distinctive feature of Wansu is the bow in which the practitioner keeps hand and fist together. The hands are held either slightly off to one side, or in front of the chest. This is done while standing in either a Naihanchi or Seiuchin stance. Some martial artists state that this action is strictly symbolic in nature, the open hand meaning peace with the closed fist denoting a willingness to fight if need be, much the same as the traditional Isshin-ryu bow. Others maintain that this gesture is paying homage to the Chinese influences on the kata, as the open/closed hand closely resembles the salutation of some forms of Shaolin boxing.

Wansu's lineage is linked to the Shuri-te systems. It is generally believed that Takahara Pechin was in the first generation of Okinawan karate-ka to practice these movements. He later taught the form to Sakugawa, who went on to teach it to Bushi Matsumura. Matsumura was Chotoku Kyan's Shuri-te instructor, and the kata was then passed from Kyan to Shimabuku. Of all the kata's in the Isshin-ryu system, Wansu has the most varied interpretations. However, the differences between how the form is performed in Isshin-ryu and other styles are of no great magnitude.

Chinto. Chinto has one of the most colorful histories of all the Isshin-ryu kata. One story says Chinto was a shipwrecked Chinese sailor on Okinawa who was skilled in Chuan Fa. Hiding out by day, he would slip out at night and steal food from local villagers. The villagers soon grew outraged and demanded a stop be put to this behavior. The residing lord at the time sent his most trusted warrior, Pechin Matsumora, to apprehend this vagabond. Matsumora found Chinto, but each time he tried to capture the sailor, he would evade Matsumora's attack. Matsumora returned to his king and reported that this man would harm no one. Afterwards,

Matsumora sought out Chinto to ask for instructions in his martial art. Matsumora later organized the techniques into the form seen today.

This is the popular story of Chinto, but one must take into consideration that the story's original boundaries, like most fables or legends, have probably been stretched over the years. Some historians claim the story is more fiction than fact. Why, for instance, would a Chinese sailor hide from the Okinawans? The development of this form came at a time when Okinawan/Chinese relationships were very strong, and there were already several Chinese communities on Okinawa. Some claim that Chinto was actually a Chinese envoy or military attaché, much like Kusanku and Wansu. As such, it is quite probable that this gentleman from China probably instructed more people than Pechin Matsumora.

Chinto is a form with very elusive footwork. Other Isshin-ryu katas usually have one dominant stance, and the footwork tends to be 'heavy' and 'rooted' in nature. In Chinto however, the practitioner is constantly shifting their weight and body posture. It is very light and uses many transitional stances and body shifts. One of Chinto's signature movements is a double jump kick at the kata's beginning.

Kusanku. Kusanku is sometimes referred to as the 'night fighting kata.' This refers to the opening movements at the beginning of the form. This interpretation, however, can be very misleading.

The history of Kusanku is a very colorful one. Sakugawa is credited with developing this kata. The story told is that Sakugawa came upon a Chinese gentleman (Kusanku) standing on a bridge watching the water below. As a prank, Sakugawa snuck up and tried to push him off. Kusanku turned, grabbed Sakugawa's arm, and reprimanded him for what he tried to do. It was at this moment when one of Kusanku's students walked up and introduced the two, informing Kusanku that Sakugawa was a local karate-ka with great potential. Kusanku told Sakugawa that if he wanted to learn not only the "how," but also the "why" of the martial arts, he should train with him. Afterwards, Sakugawa went and told his sensei, Takahara Pechin, who advised him to study with Kusanku.

Sakugawa studied under Kusanku for a period of six to eight years before the Chinese envoy returned to China. It was at the end of his apprenticeship when Takahara, Sakugawa's first instructor, passed away. Sakugawa went on to develop the Kusanku kata utilizing techniques he learned from both Pechin and Kusanku. Sakugawa taught the form to Matsumora who later taught it to Chotoku Kyan, one of Shimabuku's instructors.

Kusanku is a very elusive kata with various slipping and side-stepping movements. It also makes use of techniques such as dropping below an opponent's attack and striking into such areas as the lower abdomen, knees, or groin. Kusanku also contains some of the softer hand movements in the Isshin-ryu system. The Kusanku and Chinto katas are regarded as two of the most complex in Shimabuku's system.

Sunsu. Sunsu, or 'strong one,' was Shimabuku's nickname. This is the only original kata in the Isshin-ryu system. It was developed by Shimabuku in his later years and contains what allegedly are some of his favorite techniques. This gives Sunsu the appearance of being the culmination of all the other katas rolled into one. Interestingly enough, some movements within the kata have a strong resemblance to forms found in other systems. For instance, Sunsu's opening movements, up to the first set of double gouges, are almost exactly the same as the opening movements used in the Tomari-te version of Seisan.

There are various theories concerning Sunsu's place in Isshin-ryu karate. As mentioned earlier, some consider the kata simply a collection of Shimabuku's favorite techniques rolled into one. Others consider it a 'summary' of the Isshin-ryu system, with all the kata leading up to Sunsu. There is validity to be found in both theories. Techniques and principles found in the Sunsu kata are, in fact, drawn from all aspects of the Isshin-ryu system—from the charts, to Seisan, to Kusanku, and additional techniques found nowhere else. Some practitioners state that Sunsu is the final progression in empty-handed kata development. Once a practitioner hits this level, some believe the only two kata that need to be practiced are Sanchin and Sunsu.

Sunsu contains almost all the elements of movement that are present in the other katas. There are slipping, shifting, side-stepping, linear, and even circular movements. Unlike many of the katas that can be pigeonholed as 'soft' or 'hard,' the same can not be said for Sunsu. Its movements are so diversified that it is almost impossible to classify.

Whatever one's views on Sunsu are, one thing is certain—the kata can be considered Tatsuo Shimabuku's signature on Isshin-ryu karate. These are the teachings of a man who reached the highest levels of development in the martial arts. The form is drawn from his years of experience, and from his own evolution and progression as a karate-ka.

CHAPTER 12

The Practice of Kata

"Pay your respects to Buddha, but never honor him." That was a saying I learned from one of my first instructors. It always comes to mind when I hear people talk of kata and their value in different systems. Kata is perhaps one of the most common means of training in the martial arts. The importance of forms differs from system to system. If you visited a school that emphasized kickboxing, the practice of kata would not be stressed as much as it would in a Tai Chi school. Some practitioners say forms help develop aspects of one's martial art that would otherwise remain neglected. Other practitioners disagree, stating that forms are too binding and do not allow any room for personal development.

In the earlier years of Okinawan karate, kata was the main method of practicing. This was done not only to preserve technique, but also to ensure that the practitioners did not harm each other. It should be emphasized that prior to 1920, karate had no sport or competitive aspects to it. Okinawan karate had no point sparring matches. It was strictly an art of combat, and the techniques were designed and practiced to inflict maximum damage. Times have changed however, and today, perhaps due to the growth of sport karate, the goal of many techniques is not to inflict damage, but to score points in refereed matches. In this type of environment, the principles stressed in kata are of little or no importance. The question we must now answer is, where does this leave us with regards to practicing forms?

In keeping with the spirit of competition, kata also has kept up with the sport karate circuits. Kata competitions are held alongside point sparring matches, and participants are judged on their execution of the form, their technique, focus, and things of this nature. In many instances the practitioner may have modified his form for competition and made it more acrobatic than it originally was. Some even develop their own forms specifically for tournaments. While many of the competitors in karate tournaments are fine *athletes*, we must consider the ramifications 'tournament training' has on a student's development as a *martial artist*.

In many of today's sport-oriented business dojos, kata is often used to promote students within the school. In many cases, prospective students will enroll in a course that guarantees them promotion after they learn a certain number of forms and attend class a certain number of times per week. These courses require students to learn many techniques within a given time and it would not be out of place to say that more emphasis is placed on completing "requirements" rather then actual development as martial artists. Many students in these types of schools are (unknowingly) learning a quasi-martial art where relations between student and instructor are of a corporate nature. This is often disguised by an instructor's attempts at instilling what is assumed to be a 'traditional' environment by requiring Japanese, Chinese, or Korean be spoken in class. The bottom line is that students are learning how to acquire rank and not learning how to be a martial artist.

In contrast, there are other schools that emphasize kata as the backbone of all development and training. The practitioner's whole process is influenced and controlled by his development in forms. This type of training can be found in many of the hard line traditional karate dojos, and is also found in many of the internal systems of fighting. Many practitioners of Tai Chi, for instance, base their development upon form practice, with many systems of Tai Chi revolving around a particular form, either a long or short version which can take the practitioner anywhere from five to twenty-five minutes to complete.

In many schools, karate dojos in particular, the student is required to learn not only the kata, but its history as well. In a good number of these schools, kata is all-encompassing, with the practice of self-defense techniques and kumite executed exactly as they appear in kata. This type of training is commonly found in Japanese or Okinawan karate dojos. Kata is stressed daily and on many occasions group workouts will consist of kata practices where the whole class executes kata in time to the instructor's cadence. During these workouts, uniformity in performance is stressed with one practitioner's execution of kata varying little from the next, regardless of body stature.

Because of this type of training, it is not uncommon for the student to take on the movements of his or her instructor. The student naturally thinks that his instructor represents the 'only' way of practice. Students are usually not taught different techniques or taught how the kata can be customized for their own body type. Student's mimicking their instructor and not being taught any other way to perform kata only detracts from the student's creativity and produces clones of the instructor as opposed to developing martial artists.

As with many things, the solution seems to lie in the balance. The teachers that use kata to help develop the practitioner both mentally and physically usually end up with students who have a strong grasp of kata but have also maintained their own individuality and sense of creativity. This type of instructor may drill kata initially, but as the student progresses, use it as a springboard to help the student evolve into what could be deemed a complete martial artist. The student has a solid foundation in the arts, but has also utilized his own creativity in helping develop a method of training that enabled him to explore and create his own identity as a martial artist.

Isshin-ryu's kata contain most, if not all, of the system's major techniques, principles, philosophies and tactics. The basis for teaching Isshin-ryu today lays primarily in the teaching of its formal kata from instructor to student. It is not uncommon, however, to find schools which disregard the practice of kata entirely. Instead they prefer to deal with what they consider to be the real issue of fighting—training in the ring, practicing, and perfecting point kumite methods. Often, students from schools that train in this manner prove to be excellent tournament competitors, but know very little about true combative technique. It could be argued that what they are learning is nothing more than techniques designed to win a very aggressive form of tag. It should be noted here that point fighting should *not* be confused with other methods of full-contact fighting such as Thai kickboxing. Thai and other full-contact fighters train in their respective arts for years and usually perfect not only sport, but also combative skills without the aid of kata.

After examining the various thoughts on the importance of kata, we are still left with the question of what role it plays in Isshin-ryu. Is kata the bottomless pit of knowledge from which all our answers about the martial arts will come? The answer is no. If anything is to be considered a bottomless pit of knowledge, it should be our own insights and creativity, with kata as the guideline that will lead us toward the knowledge we seek.

CHAPTER 13

Stances and Footwork
of Isshin-Ryu

Like most systems of Okinawan karate, Isshin-ryu is basically practiced as a linear method of fighting which utilizes
circular hand movements. "Linear" however may not accurately describe Isshin-ryu in its more advanced stages, as it might
cause one to overlook the style's angular body shifting and
slipping methods that are used throughout the system.

Japanese karate unlike Okinawan karate is today influenced
not only by Okinawan systems of Te but also by the Japanese
methods of Budo and Bujutsu, where as Okinawan karate is
heavily influenced by Chinese systems of fighting. This is evident in not only technique but also footwork, with some styles
of Japanese karate adopting methods of movement from
Japanese Budo and Bujutsu. In contrast, the Okinawan forms
of karate have a tendency to retain their earlier Chinese influences. When comparing Japanese and Okinawan karate foot
work, the contrasts are very significant in some aspects, while
in others there is very little contrast between the two.

Isshin-ryu has seven major stances. They are Seisan,
Seiuchin, Naihanchi, Sanchin, T, and Reversed T. Some methods of teaching also utilize the Musubi stance. Isshin-ryu utilizes all its stances in a multipurpose role that allows for much
diversity in technique. However, many practitioners consider
the workhorse of Isshin-ryu to be Seisan.

Seiuchin, or horse stance, is also another workhorse stance
used much in the same fashion as Seisan. Seiuchin is usually
employed in linear and angular modes. Its strong points are
close range and grappling scenarios, where a low center of
gravity is required.

The Reversed T and T stances, which are also known as
'cat stances' are not utilized by most practitioners as much as
the Seisan and Seiuchin stances are. These two stances are pri-

marily transitional movements that are excellent when used for covering distance, side-stepping, or when used in any form of slipping or circular maneuvers. Of all the stances in Isshin-ryu, the utilization of the cat stances is probably the most neglected system wide. This is due to many misconceptions as to the role they play in Isshin-ryu's footwork.

The role of the Sanchin stance is also very misconceived by many Isshin-ryu practitioners. The Sanchin stance's main role in Isshin-ryu is considered by many to be a training device. However, the stance can be utilized in combative fashion as is done in Goju-ryu. In Isshin-ryu, the Sanchin stance's major form of utilization is within the Sanchin kata where dynamic tension is stressed. Sanchin is an inward-gripping stance that helps the practitioner develop power from the ground up. Along with the dropping of one's center into the lower abdominal region, it also strengthens muscular groups in the legs, and teaches the practitioner how to gain more control over his *hara* or abdominal region.

Naihanchi is another stance that is sometimes considered more of a training tool. Its application however in combative modes is used through out Isshin-ryu, particularly in close quarter scenarios or where slipping and or shifting of the body's position is required. Naihanchi is traditionally thought of as stance suited for sideways fighting. Although it can be utilized in such a fashion at close ranges in a linear mode, maneuverability is greatly sacrificed at any other range of combat. Like Sanchin, Naihanchi is also an inward-gripping stance which is used by many Shuri-te systems of Okinawan karate to develop the practitioner's leg and lower abdominal regions in much the same fashion as Naha-te karate-ka utilize Sanchin.

The Musubi stance is used by some Isshin-ryu dojo in kata performance, usually Seisan, In other Isshin-ryu schools it is not recognized as a formal stance. The use of the Musubi stance is one of a transitional mode for quick-shifting movements where speed, not power, takes precedence. In some versions of the Seisan kata, it is utilized in this manner during execution of the 'bridge of nose' technique backfist, depending upon how the kata is practiced.

Some people may disagree with the analysis of the above mentioned stances. Keep in mind that all stances can be used in any mode the practitioner wishes. This analysis, however, is based upon the most effective method of utilizing them. Although many practitioners will favor one stance of posture over another, there is really no perfect stance in the martial arts. All stances have their strong points and all have their limitations. Like most techniques however, much of a stance's effectiveness depends upon the individual.

Many people associate stances and footwork as one in the same. This is correct to some degree. Stances or postures, simply put, are the positioning of the feet and body in a specific manner that allows the practitioner to perform certain movements or functions.

Unlike in Hollywood movies, stances are not stationary positions designed for the practitioner to move or fight out of. Instead, the practitioner should move or fight through them in one continuous flowing motion.

Footwork is the combined use of all stances in a continuous flowing movement. This practice enables the martial artist to execute various combinations of techniques and body movements in an instant, utilizing each posture to its maximum effectiveness. When it is no longer applicable to the situation, good footwork allows the practitioner to quickly switch to another posture. This action can be performed literally hundreds of times during the course of an engagement with three, four, or even five stances being moved through in a few seconds.

In many cases footwork will be the key to a system or fighter's effectiveness. Without mobility, you cannot engage an opponent in an efficient manner. It is not uncommon to see a system's foundation, principles and strategies revolve around its footwork. For instance in Aikido, without proper footwork, the dynamic sphere principle that is so crucial to this system would be very hard, if not impossible, to execute. In many instances, footwork is a crucial element for helping establish a system's identity with the view that technique is almost secondary to footwork. Many principles and tactics of a fighting art develop from the ground up. Without a stable base, there is no power or movement. However, with proper footwork beneath the practitioner, power, mobility, and grace are all present.

CHAPTER 14

Is the Past our Prologue? Have We Blindly Chosen Our Own Destiny?

During the earlier part of this century, many of the martial art masters began to reevaluate the martial arts and the purpose they serve in modern society. There were no wars to be fought and no need to practice at night for fear of Japanese soldiers discovering what was going on. The arts gradually became a tool for spiritual development or discipline to be used not purely for combat, but also as a tool to help resolve one's inner conflict, nourish one's inner self, and help the practitioner live more peacefully and meaningfully.

It was Higashionna and Itosu who began the process of transforming the Okinawan fighting arts into more than just implements of combat. Their teachings and philosophies had great impact upon Gichin Funakoshi, founder of Shotokan. As noted earlier, after he left Okinawa for the Japanese mainland, he helped change the ideogram for *kara,* which originally meant 'China,' to one meaning 'empty.' The emptiness he referred to was the need to purge one's soul and inner self from all egotistical tendencies and desire. Higashionna, Itosu, and Funakoshi were attempting to turn the emphasis of karate away from combat to one of self-discipline and development. Combat was to take more of a secondary position and what was originally Karate-jutsu became Karate-do.

Not all Okinawan practitioners agreed with this new philosophical outlook. In fact, there was much outcry against changing the ideogram, and an even greater protest over Karate-jutsu being turned into a Do form. One of the reasons for Okinawans displeasure may have been the path that the Japanese Budo were taking. Many Okinawan karate-ka looked at the Budo as nothing more than sporting events that paled in comparison to the original combative arts. These hard-core karate men did not want to see the arts of Okinawa take the same path as the modern Budo forms. They did not want their arts, arts that had a rich history of combat, become mere sport.

One must wonder if what happened on Okinawa will happen in America. Is the past always an accurate reflection of things to come? This is an especially important question today because, unlike the early practitioners on Okinawa, much more is at stake than just the switch in basic philosophical principles. Donn F. Draeger is perhaps the most well known writer on the martial arts in the United States. He was a U.S. Marine Corps officer, a martial artist of the highest caliber, held expert ranking in many arts, lived in Japan most of his life, and his writings are well known among all serious martial artists. He was one of the first to draw a distinction between a Budo ("classical martial ways of self-perfection") and a Bujutsu ("classical martial arts of self-preservation"). He's said that the ranking of priorities in modern Budo are (1) morals, (2) discipline, (3) aesthetic form. For the older Bujutsu, in contrast, the emphasis was (1) combat, (2) discipline, (3) morals. Karate, Judo, Aikido, Kempo, and other more 'modern' arts developed from older forms of fighting in a time when warriors fought to the death with swords and armor. What has become obvious is that practicing a martial art in America today is either for competition or to satisfy one's ego by gaining rank. If a person's primary goal is self-development or self-defense, they may have trouble finding an appropriate dojo.

The martial arts in America have become much the same as major league sports. We've allowed ourselves to become commercialized, franchised, and incorporated. Money has taken the place of ethics and training is now something to be sold. It doesn't matter if the product is effective or not, more important is the image that is put forth. It is this image that allows the customer the satisfaction of being able to state, "Yes, I take karate" or, "Yes, I am a black belt."

More and more, we are alienating the martial arts from society. The arts are rapidly evolving into sporting contests and much of the training done today doesn't possess the depth or mental scope required to achieve the mindset Funakoshi spoke of when he stressed emptiness. Today's frame of mind is to excel, to win an event. There is no doubt that much of the training done is very physically demanding, yet many of the techniques utilized are for sporting events. They would have very little effect if used in a combative confrontation. The real flaw is that the martial arts have been exploited so much and for so long in America that we have lost the ability to grasp what is real philosophically, what isn't, what techniques will work, and what won't. With very few exceptions, our ranking structures and political organizations are more concerned with organizing tournaments and not the development of an individual. It does not matter if a practitioner has been involved in the martial arts thirty years. If this person walks into a tournament without that coveted black, or red and white belt around their waist, they will more than likely find themselves on the sidelines instead of their expertise being called upon to help officiate.

It is no small wonder that many of the older, more legitimate and true martial practitioners are keeping a low profile and instructing a handful of students in some out of the way place where the word 'tournament' is seldom spoken of seriously.

Tournaments or martial festivals are not new to the Okinawan karate systems or any other martial art. Even today there are some exceptional tournaments which are truly martial in nature. This "age of glitter" is unfortunately here to stay. One thing for certain is that the individuals who do want to experience martial teachings will seek out an appropriate instructor. When they find them and begin to practice in a true martial manner, it may seem almost alien in nature initially. For those who persevere however, they'll find that what they are doing is head and shoulders above the rest of crowd. They'll begin to recognize what true martial arts are.

I read a book written by a somewhat famous, very colorful Army officer with many wars and years of experience behind him to draw on. He said that if he could have his way, there would be two separate armies. The first would be an Army whose training was geared for showmanship, who executed parade ground maneuvers flawlessly, who dressed in bright shiny uniforms and guarded the palace. They would travel all over the country giving demonstrations of close-order drills. This is the unit that would always be present when visiting dignitaries were on hand. The second Army would not be brought before the public's eye. It would not be concerned with aesthetics. It would be a fighting force, dressed in jungle fatigues, and consist of a small elite unit of highly motivated individuals skilled in all aspects warfare who thought no mission or battle too difficult to take on. Their training would be of a completely martial nature and focused on how to take out the enemy as quickly and efficiently as possible.

This statement, extreme as it may be, accurately reflects the current division in the martial arts in America today. On one hand we have Hollywood, and the sport-oriented methods with all their flash. Due to the media being everywhere and anywhere, this is the side of the martial arts that most people see and what most people base their opinions of the martial arts on. Then there are those who practice in order to reap the benefits of personal development and evolution. These are the practitioners whom the public's eye very seldom falls upon. If an instructor of this ilk does get noticed, the public is usually at a loss for understanding. "Where are all the trophies, colored belts, ribbons, flying side kicks, and flaming board breaking demonstrations?" they may wonder. It may certainly be cliché, but only time will tell how these two very different trains of thought will continue to evolve and develop.

The past in many cases is our prologue, and this is especially true with the martial arts in today's society. Prior to the Okinawans taking a more philosophical attitude towards their martial arts, many Japanese Bujutsu practitioners of the day were expressing their displeasure with Budo systems in existence at the time. Many considered the Budo forms to be nothing more than shallow imitations even though the systems of Budo in that era held more of a martial attitude than what is to be found today in many systems of modern day karate.

One hundred years ago, no one could have imagined the impact that modern day systems of Japanese Budo, and the transformation of Okinawan karate into a Do system, would have on the world. Combining martial arts with American's penchant for quick results, capital gains, and "bigger is better attitudes," the martial art scene in the states has progressed to create an out of control, martial Frankenstein. The aims and results of many martial arts in America have become so distorted that even if an individual wished to partake in the study of a Budo form, or any other martial art for its intended purpose, it would almost seem to be an impossible undertaking.

The history of the martial arts is filled with festivals and martial oriented sporting events where practitioners were allowed to come and show their abilities. The serious practice of a martial art encompasses spiritual, physical, combative, and even sport oriented aspects, but all should be stressed in equal quantities. Other societies, for instance, have successfully managed to balance both the sporting and martial aspects of the arts. For instance, Thai kickboxing has long been considered a national sport in Southeast Asia, yet the art is also martial in nature and complete with its own traditions, history, and symbolism.

In recent years many have tried to restore an air of traditionalism about the martial arts by imposing such rules as white gi's only at tournaments, requiring members of the training hall to bow from a kneeling position, and by requiring other traditional mannerisms. The list goes on and on, yet what is being overlooked by these so-called staunch traditionalists is what the *essence* of their training should be about. Window dressing such as bowing and wearing white gi's will not make a martial artist if his motivating factor for practice is the satisfaction of his own ego through sport oriented competition. In the book *Modern Budo & Bujutsu*, Draeger quotes Okakura Kakuzo who had this to say about the Japanese Budo prior to his death in 1913:

> *The machinery of competition imposes the monotony of fashion instead of the variety of life. The cheap is worshiped in place of the beautiful, while the rush and struggle of modern existence give no opportunity for the leisure required for the crystallization of ideals.*

For many of us Okakura Kakuzo's quote is one well worth considering.

CHAPTER 15

Isshin-Ryu—Its Function in Today's Society

This chapter could have easily been devoted to the American martial arts community as a whole, but since this text's focus is upon Isshin-ryu, we will explore its function within today's society.

Our society as a whole is consumer oriented. It is a society in which labels are very important for establishment of one's self-image and the image that others may form of us. Many forms of positive reinforcement in American society are measured by the awards given or titles granted. In many cases it doesn't matter if an individual is very proficient at a certain task or endeavor. If he doesn't have a title *stating* this, then he may not be heard or respected by others.

Every martial art is influenced by the society it comes from and the society it is transplanted into. This proves especially true for the martial arts within America today. Today a karate-ka's progress is usually measured in rank held and trophies won. Within today's sport karate society, awards establish the karate-ka's identity to not only their fellow martial artists, but to themselves as well. Tournaments do not necessarily measure a karate-ka's proficiency as a martial artist, but they do help establish his identity in the competitive arena and serve as means of positive reinforcement for the individual. Although this one-dimensional approach neglects many other aspects that can be attained through the martial arts, our society places a great deal of importance on public recognition.

Our society and cultural mores have enabled many people to become quite successful in their chosen fields. It could be argued that independence, freedom, healthy competition, and the motivation it creates are some of the ideals that have helped the United States become a world power. On the other hand it also ingrains in the average American that to pursue an endeavor with no tangible rewards is a waste of time. To pursue a task purely for self-development without the slightest hint of recognition is not a worthy one. If tournaments, trophies, ribbons, and belts were to be eliminated from the martial arts scene tomorrow, there is no doubt that a tremendous number of people would drop out of sight. To endlessly pursue an endeavor like the martial arts where there is no end in sight requires an individual to develop a different mindset, one contrary to today's society. This mindset requires patience, development of analytical and creative resources, as well as a strong will. All of these concepts, when applied to one's daily life, can greatly enhance it.

CHAPTER 16

Evolution and
Our Future

In many instances throughout this book, the word "Isshin-ryu" could have been substituted for many other systems. Isshin-ryu's development and current status in America parallels that of many other systems of martial arts. All martial artists are on a journey of personal evolution. Regardless of whether the practitioner studies Tai Chi, Aikido, Bando, or Shotokan, evolution begins from day one of practice and is a process we all go through.

During the study of martial arts, one is constantly developing, changing, refining, and evolving. In many cases, what the student learned on the first day has, by the third year, been dissected, reconstructed, and practiced in a manner which bears only slight resemblance to what was taught originally. After some years of change, experimentation, evolution, and refinements this same student may be surprised to find his technique drifting back to the simplicity of the techniques taught during his first few days of study. His path has ended where it first began, and a new path that promises further physical and mental development now presents itself to the seasoned practitioner.

Some reject this theory of experimentation and evolution. They stay strictly with the principles and techniques they feel are the essence of *their* system. For them, to be branded a system's practitioner means only executing and utilizing prescribed techniques and principles in their style. What they may not see however, is that practicing with blinders on, and allowing themselves to be bound by style, limits their own development as martial artists.

At its highest state of perfection, a martial system will encompass all elements of combat and individual development. During the initial stages of learning though, elements and principles are isolated and presented to the student as the systems core. In actuality, this only serves to establish a base for the student to build upon. Once this base is established, other elements are brought to the practitioner's attention to help further his development. The martial arts are still fairly new in America. It may be in our nature to think in terms of absolutes towards the various systems and styles. It is easy to pigeonhole, classify, and quantify the various elements of different systems. This gives us the ability to say, "That is a Goju technique and this is an Aikido technique." While this might make things easier for the beginner, it will only limit the development of the more advanced practitioner. It is this sense of absolutes that keeps us from benefiting when practicing the martial arts. Thinking in this manner not only hampers our physical development, but our spiritual, social, and intellectual progress as well.

The perfection, understanding, and mastery of one's chosen style is of great importance in the development of a practitioner. Mastery of one system is extremely important. It gives the practitioner a stable base of knowledge and understanding about the martial arts and themselves. Without this solid foundation, it is easy to lose sight and perspective of one's evolution during later stages of development. This happens all too frequently and results in individual's drifting from system to system without having made an in-depth study of anyone one particular style. True growth, evolution, and development of martial artists begins *after* they have achieved an extremely high level of expertise in their chosen systems. It is at this point when they can no longer look to the system for answers—they must now look at themselves.

Looking inward is something a practitioner can do only because there is already a strong base of understanding present. Mastery of one system, the subsequent journey into oneself, and the examination of other systems is a path which leads the practitioner through many levels of learning which are not only related to combat, but to our day-to-day struggle as human beings as well.

Somewhere, for the first time, a young practitioner is putting on a brand new gi and stiff white belt. He's a little intimidated by the alien surroundings of the dojo, and his tongue twists in knots when trying to pronounce the strange words of Isshin-ryu or his chosen art. Even though he is intimidated, there is still this gleam in his eye, and thoughts of breaking boards and flying side kicks dance in his head. He steps on the dojo floor for the first time, bowing in a somewhat unsure manner, and begins.

As instructors and martial artists, it is these people—the beginners—who we should nurture. We must teach them the true meaning of the martial arts. Our instructions must be free from the political bickering and egotistical meanderings currently plaguing us. We need to teach these beginners that the martial arts are not only for self-defense, but provide us with a well-worn path toward personal development. The future of the martial arts lay in their hands, and it is up to us to show them the Way.

Afterword

It was 1976 when I first began formal martial arts lessons. After pestering my mother for several months, she finally gave in and enrolled me in the Harold Long School of Karate. Mr. Long met us at the door and escorted us into his office. He was a big man, powerfully built with a Marine crew cut, and his voice had the rasp of a drill sergeant. I would soon learn he was a strict disciplinarian who never hesitated to voice his opinion.

A few months later, I saw the movie *Kung Fu* with David Carridine. There was a distinct difference between the TV characters and the real ones I encountered on an almost daily basis. The Isshin-ryu pioneers such as Mr. Long could be humble and mysterious at times. They could also be headstrong, swaggering, and even arrogant. They were tough men who, as young Marines, had gone to war in places like Inchon, the Chosun reservoir, Hue, and Khe Sanh. Put any two of these men together and a heated debate would inevitably erupt about the true way to teach Isshin-ryu.

If we put their differences aside for a moment, we see that all of these men had three things in common: (1) An unyielding devotion to Tatsuo Shimabuku. (2) An abundance of self-confidence. (3) No illusions about what fighting or combat were. What they didn't understand, they made up for with determination. What they lacked in skill or insight was compensated for by sheer fighting prowess.

It is easy for the younger generation to dwell in the lore that surrounds these early pioneers. It is even easier to look back and judge a generation that we did not grow up in. These men were certainly not saints, and some were more qualified to teach than others were. Some had feats that will never be surpassed, while others had students that surpassed them. What they *all* had however, was a determination and drive to teach and pass on the principles of Isshin-ryu. They believed in the system, brought back what they learned, and did the best with what they had. Most importantly, they instilled the spirit of martial arts into the lives of those they touched. It is for this we should be extremely thankful.

Bibliography

Armstrong, Steve. *Seisan Kata of Isshinryu Karate.* Ohara Publication, 1973.

Corcoran, John and Farkas, Emil. *The Original Martial Arts Encyclopedia: Tradition-History-Pioneers.* Pro Action Publishing, 1993.

Demura, Fumio. *Bo: Karate Weapon of Self Defense.* Ohara, 1976.

Demura, Fumio. *Nunchaku: Karate Weapon of Self Defense.* Ohara, 1971.

Demura, Fumio. *Sai: Karate Weapon of Self Defense.* Ohara, 1971.

Draeger, Donn F. and Smith, Robert W. *Asian Fighting Arts,* Tokyo: Kodansha International Ltd., 1969

Draeger, Donn F. *Modern Bujutsu & Budo,* Weatherhill, 1974.

Draeger, Donn F. *Classical Budo: Martial Arts and Ways of Japan.* Weatherhill, 1973.

Draeger, Donn F. *Classical Bujutsu: Martial Arts and Ways of Japan.* Weatherhill, 1983.

Funakoshi, Gichin. *Karate-Do Kyohan,* Tokyo: Kodansha International Ltd., 1973

Funakoshi, Gichin. *Karate-Do My Way of Life.* Kodansha, 1975.

Funakoshi, Gichin. *Karate-Do Nyumon.* Kodansha, 1988.

Kerr, George H. *Okinawa: The History of an Island People.* Tuttle, 1958.

Kim, Richard. *The Weaponless Warriors: An Informal History of Okinawan Karate,* Ohara, 1974.

Mattson, George E. *Uechi-Ryu Karate-Do* (Classical Chinese-Okinawan Self Defense). Peabody Publishing, 1974.

Morgan, Forrest E. *Living the Martial Way.* Barricade Books, 1992.

Musashi, Miyamoto. *A Book of Five Rings: A Guide to Strategy.* The Overlook Press, 1974.

Nagamine, Shoshin. *The Essence of Okinawan Karate-Do.* (Shorin-Ryu). Tuttle, 1979.

Orlando, Bob. *Martial Arts America: A Western Approach to Eastern Arts.* Frog Ltd., 1997.

Ratti, Oscar and Westbrook, Adele. *Secrets of the Samurai: A Survey of the Martial Arts of Feudal Japan.* Tuttle, 1973.

Skoss, Diane. *Koryu Bujutsu—Classical Warrior Traditions of Japan.* Koryu Books, 1997.

Suzuki, D.T. *Zen and the Japanese Culture.* Pantheon Books, 1959.

Suzuki, Shunryu. *Zen Mind Beginners Mind.* Weatherhill, 1970.

Toguchi, Seikichi. *Okinawan Goju-Ryu: The Fundamentals of Shorei-Kan Karate.* Ohara, 1976.

Turnball, Stephen R. *The Samurai, A Military History.* Macmillan Publishing Co., 1977.

Webb, Glen. *The Manual of Isshinryu Karate.* Self Published. 1976.

Yamaguchi, Gosei. *The Fundamentals of Goju-Ryu Karate.* Ohara, 1972.

Yang, Jwing-Ming. *The Essence of Shaolin White Crane: Martial Power and Qigong.* YMAA Publication Center, 1996.

Index

BOOKS FROM YMAA

6 HEALING MOVEMENTS
101 REFLECTIONS ON TAI CHI CHUAN
108 INSIGHTS INTO TAI CHI CHUAN — A STRING OF PEARLS
A WOMAN'S QIGONG GUIDE
ADVANCING IN TAE KWON DO
ANCIENT CHINESE WEAPONS
ANALYSIS OF SHAOLIN CHIN NA 2ND ED.
ARTHRITIS RELIEF — CHINESE QIGONG FOR HEALING &
    PREVENTION, 3RD ED.
BACK PAIN RELIEF — CHINESE QIGONG FOR HEALING & PREVENTION
    2ND ED
BAGUAZHANG
CARDIO KICKBOXING ELITE
CHIN NA IN GROUND FIGHTING
CHINESE FAST WRESTLING — THE ART OF SAN SHOU KUAI JIAO
CHINESE FITNESS — A MIND / BODY APPROACH
CHINESE TUI NA MASSAGE
COMPLETE CARDIOKICKBOXING
COMPREHENSIVE APPLICATIONS OF SHAOLIN CHIN NA
DR. WU'S HEAD MASSAGE—ANTI-AGING AND HOLISTIC HEALING
    THERAPY
EIGHT SIMPLE QIGONG EXERCISES FOR HEALTH, 2ND ED.
ESSENCE OF SHAOLIN WHITE CRANE
ESSENCE OF TAIJI QIGONG, 2ND ED.
EXPLORING TAI CHI
FIGHTING ARTS
INSIDE TAI CHI
KATA AND THE TRANSMISSION OF KNOWLEDGE
LIUHEBAFA FIVE CHARACTER SECRETS
MARTIAL ARTS ATHLETE
MARTIAL ARTS INSTRUCTION
MARTIAL WAY AND ITS VIRTUES
MEDITATIONS ON VIOLENCE
MIND/BODY FITNESS — A MIND / BODY APPROACH
MUGAI RYU — THE CLASSICAL SAMURAI ART OF DRAWING THE
    SWORD
NATURAL HEALING WITH QIGONG — THERAPEUTIC QIGONG
NORTHERN SHAOLIN SWORD, 2ND ED.
OKINAWA'S COMPLETE KARATE SYSTEM — ISSHIN RYU
POWER BODY
PRINCIPLES OF TRADITIONAL CHINESE MEDICINE
QIGONG FOR HEALTH & MARTIAL ARTS 2ND ED.
QIGONG FOR LIVING

QIGONG FOR TREATING COMMON AILMENTS
QIGONG MASSAGE —FUNDAMENTAL TECHNIQUES FOR HEALTH AN
    RELAXATION, 2ND ED.
QIGONG MEDITATION — EMBRYONIC BREATHING
QIGONG MEDITATION—SMALL CIRCULATION
QIGONG, THE SECRET OF YOUTH
QUIET TEACHER
ROOT OF CHINESE QIGONG, 2ND ED.
SHIHAN TE — THE BUNKAI OF KATA
SUNRISE TAI CHI
SURVIVING ARMED ASSAULTS
TAEKWONDO — ANCIENT WISDOM FOR THE MODERN WARRIOR
TAE KWON DO — THE KOREAN MARTIAL ART
TAEKWONDO — SPIRIT AND PRACTICE
TAO OF BIOENERGETICS
TAI CHI BOOK
TAI CHI CHUAN — 24 & 48 POSTURES
TAI CHI CHUAN MARTIAL APPLICATIONS, 2ND ED.
TAI CHI CONNECTIONS
TAI CHI DYNAMICS
TAI CHI SECRETS OF THE ANCIENT MASTERS
TAI CHI SECRETS OF THE WU & LI STYLES
TAI CHI SECRETS OF THE WU STYLE
TAI CHI SECRETS OF THE YANG STYLE
TAI CHI THEORY & MARTIAL POWER, 2ND ED.
TAI CHI WALKING
TAIJI CHIN NA
TAIJI SWORD, CLASSICAL YANG STYLE
TAIJIQUAN, CLASSICAL YANG STYLE
TAIJIQUAN THEORY OF DR. YANG, JWING-MING
THE CROCODILE AND THE CRANE
THE CUTTING SEASON
THE WAY OF KATA—A COMPREHENSIVE GUIDE TO DECIPHERING
    MARTIAL APPS.
THE WAY OF KENDO AND KENJITSU
THE WAY OF SANCHIN KATA
THE WAY TO BLACK BELT
TRADITIONAL CHINESE HEALTH SECRETS
TRADITIONAL TAEKWONDO—CORE TECHNIQUES, HISTORY, AND
    PHILOSOPHY
WILD GOOSE QIGONG
WISDOM'S WAY
XINGYIQUAN, 2ND ED.

DVDS FROM YMAA

ANALYSIS OF SHAOLIN CHIN NA
BAGUAZHANG 1,2, & 3 —EMEI BAGUAZHANG
CHEN STYLE TAIJIQUAN
CHIN NA IN DEPTH COURSES 1 — 4
CHIN NA IN DEPTH COURSES 5 — 8
CHIN NA IN DEPTH COURSES 9 — 12
EIGHT SIMPLE QIGONG EXERCISES FOR HEALTH
FIVE ANIMAL SPORTS
THE ESSENCE OF TAIJI QIGONG
QIGONG MASSAGE—FUNDAMENTAL TECHNIQUES FOR HEALTH AND
    RELAXATION
SHAOLIN KUNG FU FUNDAMENTAL TRAINING 1&2
SHAOLIN LONG FIST KUNG FU — BASIC SEQUENCES
SHAOLIN SABER — BASIC SEQUENCES
SHAOLIN STAFF — BASIC SEQUENCES
SHAOLIN WHITE CRANE GONG FU BASIC TRAINING 1&2
SIMPLE QIGONG EXERCISES FOR ARTHRITIS RELIEF
SIMPLE QIGONG EXERCISES FOR BACK PAIN RELIEF
SIMPLIFIED TAI CHI CHUAN
SUNRISE TAI CHI
SUNSET TAI CHI
TAI CHI CONNECTIONS
TAI CHI ENERGY PATTERNS

TAIJI BALL QIGONG COURSES 1&2—16 CIRCLING AND 16 ROTATIN
    PATTERNS
TAIJI BALL QIGONG COURSES 3&4—16 PATTERNS OF WRAP-
    COILING & APPLICATIONS
TAIJI MARTIAL APPLICATIONS — 37 POSTURES
TAIJI PUSHING HANDS 1&2—YANG STYLE SINGLE AND DOUBLE
    PUSHING HANDS
TAIJI PUSHING HANDS 3&4—MOVING SINGLE AND DOUBLE PUSHIN
    HANDS
TAIJI SABER — THE COMPLETE FORM, QIGONG & APPLICATIONS
TAIJI & SHAOLIN STAFF - FUNDAMENTAL TRAINING
TAIJI YIN YANG STICKING HANDS
TAIJIQUAN CLASSICAL YANG STYLE
TAIJI SWORD, CLASSICAL YANG STYLE
UNDERSTANDING QIGONG 1 — WHAT IS QI? • HUMAN QI CIRCULATOR
    SYSTEM
UNDERSTANDING QIGONG 2 — KEY POINTS • QIGONG BREATHING
UNDERSTANDING QIGONG 3 — EMBRYONIC BREATHING
UNDERSTANDING QIGONG 4 — FOUR SEASONS QIGONG
UNDERSTANDING QIGONG 5 — SMALL CIRCULATION
UNDERSTANDING QIGONG 6 — MARTIAL QIGONG BREATHING
WHITE CRANE HARD & SOFT QIGONG

more products available from...
YMAA Publication Center, Inc. 楊氏東方文化出版中心
1-800-669-8892 • ymaa@aol.com • www.ymaa.com

Printed in the USA
CPSIA information can be obtained
at www.ICGtesting.com
JSHW082213140824
68134JS00014B/594